LYME
DISEASE

THE
TERRORIST
WITHIN

BY

GORDON A. GILKES MD, MPH

ISBN: 1-4392-0154-4
ISBN-13: 9781439201541

BOOK OUTLINE

PART ONE
PROFILE OF A TERRORIST BACTERIUM

1

2

3

4

5

6

PART TWO
THE LYME NETWORK

PART THREE
THE MEDICAL 'INTELLIGENCE' ON LYME

12

13

14

15

Author's note and disclaimer:

PART ONE

PROFILE OF A
TERRORIST BACTERIUM

1

AUTHOR'S INTRODUCTION

AUTHOR'S INTRODUCTION

ⅩⅩ ⅩⅩ ⅩⅩ

From 1985-1995 I ran an Urgent & Routine Medical Clinic (URMC) in which I was the chief physician with occasional help from medical colleagues in my area. It was the only such clinic in Paradise, a growing town in the beautiful hills of Northern California. I had previously served as an emergency room physician for the local hospital as well as for a hospital in Oroville, CA. where I had worked along with fellow physicians who had initiated a regular emergency patient care program in the nearby Oroville Community Hospital. From there I worked at the Redding Community Hospital and after awhile, was the head physician of the doctors who worked in the same department. I have never forgotten the long hours involved in taking care of cuts, bruises, cardiac problems, convulsing patients, and sick children. Then there was the train accident just outside of the town when I had to spend 72 hours (with very little sleep) triaging and taking care of scores of injured passengers. Those were the "good old days"? Things have changed a great deal since those days! Now we have so much uptodate electronic equipment and diagnostic availability that ER programs run smoother, and patient care is markedly improved. My last few years of Emergency medicine were spent at the Feather River Hospital before they totally renovated the ER and have become highly modernized and able to take care of vastly more complicated cases than in former times. Their services are highly respected by all those who have been through their doors.

During my time at the URMC, I came in contact with many patients who were suffering from strange symptoms which they attributed to chronic fatigue. They complained that they were simply too tired to hold down a steady job. I would refer these patients to other doctors since I was not involved in long term care.

I confess that I thought most of those "tired" patients might have been simply lazy and were probably using the disability insurance program for undeserved financial aid. Some years later, I began to experience the identical symptoms which those former patients had presented to me. This was the turning point. I was forced to change my attitude towards the symptoms those "tired" patients had complained about.

Physicians sometimes need to 'walk in their patient's shoes' before they can become genuinely sympathetic to their complaints. Because of this human 'disconnect' between patient and doctor many patients with Lyme disease have been maligned, misdiagnosed and turned away by the medical profession, sometimes by their own families and friends.

I learned from my own experience of those symptoms (fatigue, depression, weakness, an inability to work or to think properly) that they were real, not imagined. I had contracted the elusive, still often disregarded infection known as Lyme disease. But I had to travel a long and painful road before I knew for certain what it was that had attacked my normally healthy and energetic body and mind. Lyme is a ravenous disease that begins by working slowly and unobtrusively to destroy the life it touches. It is an apparently harmless intruder, lurking quietly in the human body like a terrorist awaiting an opportunity to cause havoc and finally take the life of its host.

This book contains nothing that fellow physicians may not already know or can't find in the great variety of published medical literature on Lyme disease. But I was strongly motivated, as a victim of the disease, to spend thousands of hours researching the sources which I present here in summary form for convenient reference. In doing this I am doing what I wish someone had done for me: giving you readily accessible information for your own research and investigation into the amazing and disturbing story of Lyme disease.

Today, 'the war on terror' is part of our everyday consciousness. No one doubts the very real threat of external terrorism, and there has been a global response to it. My hope is that this book will paint a convincing picture of the threat of Lyme disease so that those who read it will better understand the seriousness of the disease and its symptoms and take the necessary steps to save their health and perhaps their lives. My wish for those still skeptical health practitioners who read this book is that they will start thinking 'outside of the box' of the standard medical think tanks that so often ignore the plethora of symptoms that are regularly misdiagnosed or shrugged off (as I was once guilty of doing) as "psychological problems" and other 'waste basket' terms. We need to be aware, globally, of the dangers of another, much subtler form of terrorism exemplified by Lyme disease, the terror within.

[I am including a few pictures from the Amazon jungle in Peru for extra interest and to reduce any boredom from reading the plain text! The only non-Peruvian pic is that of my Dad whose story is featured in chapter 5. This photo was taken in England where he spent many years before immigrating to Canada where my sisters live.]

2

WHAT IS LYME DISEASE?

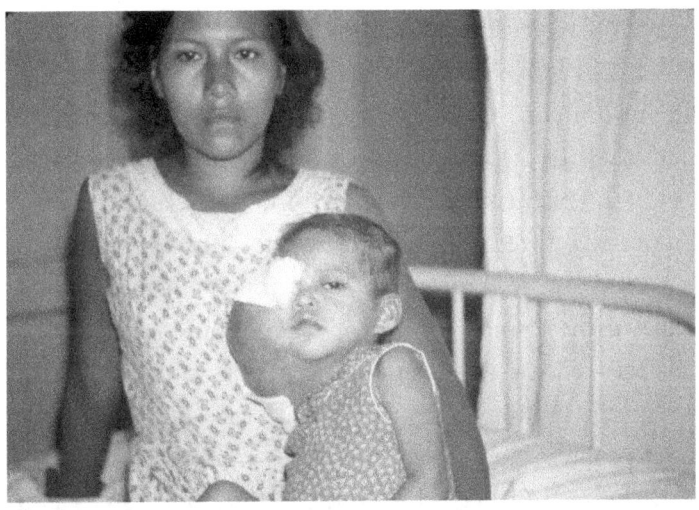

Sick child from the jungle of Peru in the clinic where the author worked, The jungle story follows later.

❁ ❁ ❁

Lyme disease was apparently first identified in the mid-1970s in Old Lyme, Connecticut, hence its name.

The origin of the disease, however, dates back more than a hundred years.

In 1883 in Breslau, Germany, a physician, Alfred Buchwald, had already recorded and described a degenerative skin disorder called acrodermatitis chronica atrophicans (ACA) This was an early footprint, as it would later turn out, of Lyme disease.

In 1909 Arvid Afzelius was fascinated by an expanding, ring-shaped skin lesion he had observed in his medical practice. Twelve years of research later he suggested that the rash came from the bite of a tiny tick with an impressive Graeco-Roman name: *Ixodes scapularis*. Another early footprint. But the real intruder's cover was still to be blown.

By the early twentieth century, links were already being discovered between the many different symptoms and signs that are now recognized as footprints of Lyme disease. Some of these were: joint problems in patients (1921), a link between the tell-tale rash and nerve problems (1922), psychiatric symptoms in patients with the rash (1930), and heart problems as well as arthritic symptoms in patients with the rash (1934). The hidden Lyme offensive – and its terrorist strategy: an attack on many fronts – had been uncovered.

In 1970 it was known, for the first time, that the deadly intruder had arrived, incognito, in the United States. Rudolph Scrimenti diagnosed and treated a patient who had been bitten by a tick while hunting grouse in Wisconsin and has, therefore, the dubious distinction of becoming Lyme's first recorded American victim.

In 1976, the first discovery of the "clustering", scatter-shot nature of this disease in the U.S. was reported by researchers at the Naval Submarine Medical Center in Southwestern Connecticut. In 1977, physician Allen Steere and his colleagues also observed this phenomenon of "clustering" when the disease was misdiagnosed as juvenile rheumatoid arthritis. They re-named the condition "Lyme arthritis" after the real culprit. But no one, it seems, was as yet aware of the true nature and origin of the disease.

In the early 1980s, an entomologist at the United States Rocky Mountain Laboratories of the National Institutes of Health, Willy Burgdorfer, M.D., Ph.D. noticed an embryonic form of parasite in the body fluid of two of the ticks he was examining. He'd read the early European researchers' findings (especially the research that had pointed to Afzelius's exotic tick, Ixodes) and decided to make a very close inspection of the tick he was investigating. He found inside the tick's stomach a group of unusually shaped, sluggish-looking, barely visible spirochetes (spiral-shaped bacteria). The spirochetes were christened *Borrelia burgdorferi* and later positively identified as the hidden agent of the mystery disease he was trying to trace.

Burgdorfer had found the source of Lyme disease : the terrorist within.

It has often been said that mankind's greatest enemies are not the large creatures of the rainforest or the oceans, though they are frequently given a bad press. There is no shortage of imagery (as in movies like "Jaws", stories of 'killer' whales, encounters with wild animals, the

"Werewolf", "Dracula" and other myths) that make wild animals seem our mortal enemies. These creatures, real or imagined, are by no means our greatest threat. That threat comes from the almost invisible presence of some of the smallest of all living creatures : disease bacteria. We are trained to be on guard against the terror that threatens us in the outside world while the *real* terror lives and breeds within our own bodies.

So how do we get Lyme disease, and what are its symptoms?

The "classical," apparently harmless, symptoms of the onset of the infection are:

1. A red rash on a small area of the skin following a tick bite.
2. The rash spreads to form a "bull's-eye" a few centimeters in diameter.
3. The rash lasts for a month or more and then goes away without any treatment.

The problem with these symptoms is that there may be no rash in 50 % or more of cases, and in many patients the rash may not be noticed because of its location on the body surface (hairy areas etc). Worse, since the infection spreads rapidly to other parts of the body, there may be other rashes that appear later. This is why the medical name for this rash is "erythema migrans". The "migrans" part of the name means that the rash can migrate to other parts of the body, appearing in different locations at different times.

So, at the outset of infection, the intruder is already mobile, opening up different 'fronts' of operation.

This may be bad news, but there's worse to come.

One of the most widespread symptoms of Lyme is – characteristically – the least likely to raise an alarm. It is a 'flu-like complaint which most of us have experienced and are familiar with. But this 'flu seems like the worst case of 'flu you ever had: it is usually accompanied by chills, fever, nausea with vomiting (though not all may have these symptoms). The illness is so debilitating that you can hardly get out of bed.

But of course there's still not enough here to ring the alarm bell.

Add back ache, neck ache as well as joint and muscle aches and you begin to suspect that this is more than 'flu. Still not enough to ring that alarm bell. The symptoms of dengué fever (for example) are similar. The problem of diagnosis gets even more difficult as we look closer.

This note is from the Canadian Lyme Disease Foundation:

"Lyme Disease symptoms may show up fast, with a bang, or very slowly and innocuously. There may be initial flu-like symptoms with fever, headache, nausea, jaw pain, light sensitivity, red eyes, muscle ache and stiff neck. Many write this off as a 'flu and because the nymph stage of the tick is so tiny many do not recall a tick bite. The classic rash may only occur or have been seen in as few as 30% of cases (many rashes in body hair and indiscrete [sic] areas go undetected). Treatment in this early stage is critical."

The good news is that some people have a reasonably easy recovery with the use of antibiotics, which if used early in the infection, and with proper dosage allows most people to recover without any serious complications.

The bad news is that, unfortunately, few people start treatment early. It's almost as if the Lyme disease agents work on the likelihood that few humans will take the early symptoms of Lyme's activity seriously. None of us wants to ring the alarm bell unless we're sure there's an emergency. It doesn't help either that these symptoms can take so many forms, appearing as 'clusters' of minor-seeming ailments. Where do we draw the line? How to decide that our symptoms are significant ?

Here is a list of symptoms: it can be found on the Canadian Lyme Foundation web site. You can download the questionnaire offered below.

As you will see, the range of operations and the variety of symptoms of this potential killer are positively dizzying.

Canadian Lyme Disease Foundation

"With symptoms present, a negative lab result means very little as they are very unreliable. The diagnosis, with today's limitations in the lab, must be clinical.

Many Lyme patients were firstly diagnosed with other illnesses such as Juvenile Arthritis, Rheumatoid Arthritis, Reactive Arthritis, Infectious Arthritis, Osteoarthritis, Fibromyalgia, Raynaud's Syndrome, Chronic Fatigue Syndrome, Interstitial Cystis, Gastroesophageal Reflux

Disease, Fifth Disease, <u>Multiple Sclerosis,</u> scleroderma, <u>Lupus,</u> <u>early ALS,</u> early <u>Alzheimers Disease,</u> <u>Crohn's disease</u>, Ménières syndrome, Sjogren's syndrome, <u>Irritable bowel syndrome,</u> Colitis, Prostatitis, <u>Psychiatric disorders</u> (bipolar, depression, etc.), encephalitis, <u>sleep disorders,</u> thyroid disease and various other illnesses.

If you have received one of these diagnoses please scroll down and see if you recognize a broader range of symptoms.

If you are a doctor please re-examine these diagnoses, incorporating Lyme in the differential diagnoses.

The one common thread with Lyme Disease is the number of systems affected - brain, central nervous system, autonomic nervous system, cardiovascular, digestive, respiratory, musculo-skeletal, etc.; and sometimes the hourly/daily/weekly/monthly changing of symptoms.

No one will have all symptoms but if many are present serious consideration must be given by any physician to Lyme as the possible culprit. Lyme is endemic in Canada period. The infection rate with Lyme in the tick population is exploding in North America and as the earth's temperature warms this trend is expected to continue.

Symptoms may come and go in varying degrees with fluctuation from one symptom to another. There may be a period of what feels like remission only to be followed by another onset of symptoms."

PRINT AND CIRCLE ALL YES ANSWERS (20 yes represents a serious potential and Lyme should be included in diagnostic workup)

Symptoms of Lyme Disease

- **<u>The Tick Bite</u> (fewer than 50% recall a tick bite or get/see the rash)**

    1. Rash at site of bite
    2. Rashes on other parts of your body
    3. Rash basically circular and spreading out (or generalized)
    4. Raised rash, disappearing and recurring

- <u>Head, Face, Neck</u>

    5. <u>Unexplained hair loss</u>
    6. Headache, mild or severe
    7. Pressure in Head
    8. Twitching of facial or other muscles
    9. Facial paralysis (<u>Bell's Palsy</u>)
    10. Tingling of nose, (tip of) tongue, cheek or <u>facial flushing</u>
    11. Stiff or painful neck
    12. Jaw pain or stiffness
    13. Dental problems (unexplained)
    14. Sore throat, clearing throat a lot, phlegm (flem), hoarseness, runny nose

- <u>Eyes/Vision</u>

    15. Double or blurry vision
    16. Increased floating spots
    17. Pain in eyes, or swelling around eyes

18. Oversensitivity to light
19. Flashing lights/Peripheral waves/phantom images in corner of eyes

- Ears/Hearing

   20. Decreased hearing in one or both ears, plugged ears
   21. Buzzing in ears
   22. Pain in ears, oversensitivity to sounds
   23. Ringing in one or both ears

- Digestive and Excretory Systems

   24. Diarrhea
   25. Constipation
   26. Irritable bladder (trouble starting, stopping) or Interstitial cystitis
   27. Upset stomach (nausea or pain) or GERD (gastroesophageal reflux disease)

- Musculoskeletal System

   28. Bone pain, joint pain or swelling, carpal tunnel syndrome
   29. Stiffness of joints, back, neck, tennis elbow
   30. Muscle pain or cramps, (Fibromyalgia)

- Respiratory and Circulatory Systems

   31. Shortness of breath, can't get full/satisfying breath, cough

32. Chest pain or rib soreness
33. Night sweats or unexplained chills
34. Heart palpitations or extra beats
35. <u>Endocarditis,</u> Heart blockage

- <u>Neurologic System</u>

36. Tremors or unexplained shaking
37. Burning or stabbing sensations in the body
38. Fatigue, <u>Chronic Fatigue Syndrome</u>, Weakness, peripheral neuropathy or partial paralysis
39. Pressure in the head
40. Numbness in body, tingling, pinpricks
41. Poor balance, dizziness, difficulty walking
42. Increased motion sickness
43. Lightheadedness, wooziness

- <u>Psychological well-being</u>

44. Mood swings, irritability, bi-polar disorder
45. Unusual depression
46. Disorientation (getting or feeling lost)
47. Feeling as if you are losing your mind
48. Over-emotional reactions, crying easily
49. Too much sleep, or insomnia
50. Difficulty falling or staying asleep
51. Narcolepsy, sleep apnea
52. Panic attacks, anxiety

- <u>Mental Capability</u>

  53. Memory loss (short or long term)
  54. Confusion, difficulty in thinking
  55. Difficulty with concentration or reading
  56. Going to the wrong place
  57. Speech difficulty (slurred or slow)
  58. Stammering speech
  59. Forgetting how to perform simple tasks

- <u>Reproduction and Sexuality</u>

  60. Loss of sex drive
  61. Sexual dysfunction
  62. Unexplained menstrual pain, irregularity
  63. Unexplained breast pain, discharge
  64. Testicular or pelvic pain

- <u>General Well-being</u>

  65. Unexplained weight gain, loss
  66. Extreme fatigue
  67. Swollen glands/lymph nodes
  68. Unexplained fevers (high or low grade)
  69. Continual infections (sinus, kidney, eye, etc.)
  70. Symptoms seem to change, come and go
  71. Pain migrates (moves) to different body parts
  72. Early on, a "flu-like" illness, after which you remain feeling unwell.

73. Low body temperature
74. Allergies/Chemical sensitivities
75. Increased effects from alcohol and possibly worse hangovers

What becomes clear amid the welter of possible signs of Lyme activity is this: multiple symptoms seem to be the standard characteristic of infestation with Lyme bacteria. These unusual 'clusters' of symptoms may not be proof of the presence of Lyme, but they should be a red flag to both patient and doctor. Further diagnosis will require a close collaboration between doctor and patient, since it will be *patient's* awareness and recording of the behaviour and effects of his or her symptoms that will help guide the doctor's research and choices of treatment. There is no simple, once-and-for-all cure for Lyme disease after it has taken hold and opened up its networks of infection.

For an even more detailed description of the signs and symptoms of Lyme click on http://cassia.org/essay.htm where you will find a very comprehensive essay by John D. Bleiweiss, M.D. on the networking ability of Lyme bacteria; *"When to Suspect Lyme Disease"*. The essay was first published in April 1994.

Here is an extract:

"There is no absolutely predictable clinical sequence for Lyme disease… The onset of complaints can not only be subtle and desultory, but delayed for a year or more.

One of my patients denied all LD related symptoms until her husband died, whereupon, a plethora of complaints cascaded into her life beginning that very day. Another had an annual flare of LD as part of an anniversary reaction centered on the date of his mother's death ... Moreover, the early constellation of symptoms can have a paucity of findings with unidimensional presentations: the onset of solitary problems such as vertigo, or recurrent upper respiratory tract infections. Over time, as the untreated LD percolates, symptoms accrue to the burgeoning clinical picture until a <u>multisystem presentation is created</u>. Other patients can have their manifold symptoms complex develop in the manner of an avalanche. These patterns represent the extremes of a clinical continuum between which there are many variations on the theme ranging from mild to severe disease. Thus, the failure of a pathognomonic (unique and specific) presentation to consistently unfold causes sufficient clinical confusion, that a punctual diagnosis is problematic. Therefore, a high index of suspicion is placed at a premium. *[i.e. the doctor may begin to suspect the patient's truthfulness]* If a clinician can't reconcile preconceived notions about how LD should announce itself with a patient's history and physical findings, it is a disservice to the patient and an abdication of professional imperatives to presumptuously conclude that the symptoms are psychosomatic or that the patient is faking!... "

... The flu-like syndrome may be absent from the initial presentation and may endure once established without treatment. Cardiac and neurologic complications can be observed sometime within the first 3 months after microbiologically contracting the disease. Arthritis (i.e. joint inflammation): distinct from arthralgias; (i.e. joint pain) can also accompany the initial clinical course, but more often develops later on between the second and sixth month from inoculation. <u>The onset of complaints can not only be subtle and desultory, but delayed for a year or</u> more.

"Many patients have symptoms intensify or reappear with physical and emotional stress, if sleep deprived, after exercise, in a hot bath, after alcohol consumption, with fasting (hypoglycemia) or dehydration. Humidity, low Barometric pressure, cold or rainy weather can elicit arthalgias, fatigue, encephalopathy or headeache."

3

CONTROVERSY, CONSPIRACY AND CONTAINMENT

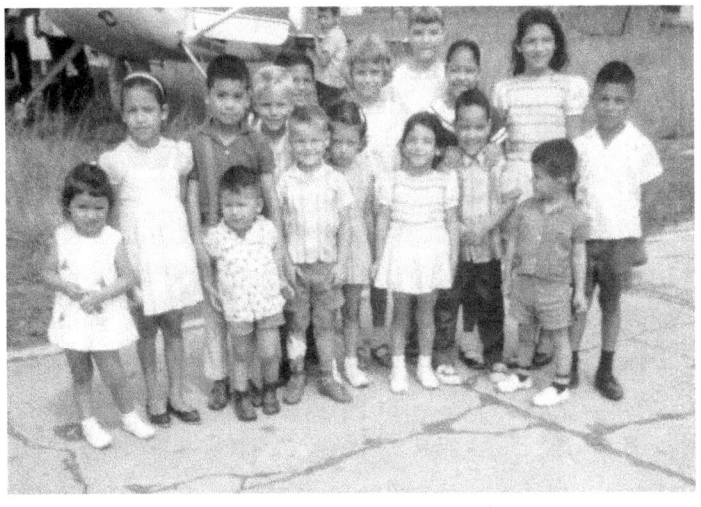

A group of healthy children in Iquitos

❦ ❦ ❦

The Controversy:

In 1983 treatment of Lyme disease began with oral and intravenous antibiotics. By 1986 the skeptics were already denying the existence of Lyme disease. As recently as March 2007, an internet publication calling itself 'Quackwatch' posted this on their website under the heading:

Lyme Disease:
Questionable Diagnosis and Treatment
by Edward McSweegan, Ph.D.

"…The fact that Lyme disease is readily curable has not discouraged the formation of over a hundred support groups and nonprofit foundations, some with ties to intravenous services, Lyme diagnostic labs, and physicians specializing in private Lyme disease practices. These groups and their ardent followers have used the Internet and other media to barrage politicians and the general public with misinformation, dire personal stories, rumors, and exaggerated claims about thousands of people being maimed, killed and bankrupted each year by Lyme disease. The core message is that Lyme is a deadly chronic disease that requires long-term antibiotic therapy paid for by insurance companies…"

The skeptics' claim (that Lyme disease had become a convenient stalking-horse for unwarranted funding and profit-making) was probably encouraged by the rapidity with which pharmaceutical companies had early begun to market 'cures' for the disease.

In 1999 a pharmaceutical company (Smith Kline Beecham) with FDA approval, put LYMErix (an unfortunate name, perhaps, with its echo of 'limericks': Lyme is no laughing matter) on the market. The new 'cure' – a genetically engineered vaccine – was widely advertised and used by thousands of Lyme sufferers. 'LYMErix' was a hit, making huge profits for the company. By 2002, after a raging controversy over the vaccine's apparently disastrous side-effects, which included arthritis and a possible resurgence of the disease with some of its worst symptoms, the vaccine was withdrawn from sale. The cure had proven to be worse than the disease, and it was removed from the marketplace. SKB , which had become SKF (Smith Kline French) by then, hadn't done enough research, it seems, and had not foreseen the human body's reaction to the protein element contained in their vaccine, nor the protean nature of the disease itself. They had rushed the troops in, so to speak, before they had properly understood the body's auto-immune reaction to their medication or the shape-shifting nature of the enemy intruder.

Pamela Weintraub, a former staff writer at Discover, former editor-in-chief of Omni Internet, and the author of 15 books on health and science, put it like this:

'In the end, the problems of LYMErix may be rooted in something far less organized than insidious - the hubris of medical science, which has sold its soul to industry for the funding it needs to survive. To be true to itself, science must acknowledge the gray areas, but to fit the needs of business, it must deal in black and white".

The skeptics remained skeptical, however, and though skepticism is often a good thing (since it puts advocacy on the defensive and promotes caution in diagnosis); it can become a stumbling block to genuine research and discovery by its refusal to remain open to the 'gray areas' of disease treatment and preventative medicine. Here is what professor McSweegan, in his article in 'Quackwatch', calls 'The Bottom Line' on Lyme disease:

- Lyme disease, when diagnosed early, is readily treatable with oral antibiotics.
- Positive antibody tests, by themselves, do not provide a sufficient basis for diagnosing Lyme disease. The diagnosis should be based on the overall clinical picture, including medical history and physical findings.
- Negative antibody testing after the first few weeks strongly suggests that the patient does not have Lyme disease.
- Many patients with chronic, nonspecific symptoms (such as headaches, fatigue, muscle aches, mental confusion, or sleep disturbances) mistakenly believe they have Lyme disease.
- Intravenous antibiotic therapy, when given appropriately, should not last more than a month. It should not be given unless oral antibiotic therapy has failed and persistent active infection has been demonstrated by culture, biopsy, or other bacteriologic technique.

- Malariotherapy, intracellular hyperthermia therapy, hyperbaric oxygen therapy, , dietary supplements, and herbs are not appropriate measures for treating Lyme disease. Doctors who recommend them should be avoided.

These magisterial statements may give the appearance of certitude, but (apart from the last two statements) they say nothing that is not already known and acknowledged in the standard medical literature about Lyme. The last two statements (except for malariotherapy) assume a certainty about treatment that is not supported by the findings of the scientific and medical research still in progress. It is extremely doubtful that medical practitioners actually treating the disease would accept these as veritable or verifiable 'truths' about Lyme disease or as best practice in its treatment. These two statements are, nevertheless, significant. *They make the common mistake of underestimating the elusive, potentially deadly nature of the enemy.*

By 2006, Lyme disease, among other tick-borne illnesses was the fastest growing infectious disease in the U.S. and the United Kingdom. Europe was already being targeted. Even countries like Brazil are seeing an increase of what they call a "Lyme-like disease" (see chapter 14)

According to the most recent estimates, there are approximately 250,000 new cases of Lyme disease in the U.S.A. each year. European countries are also seeing a huge increase. Recently the *Canadian Health Dept.* reported that more than 10,000 cases are diagnosed yearly. Some health professionals estimate the total to be at least 40,000 cases annually due to inaccurate reporting and misdiagnosis.

In an April 19th, 2006 CBC Health & Science News, Federal health officials sounded the alarm: Lyme, the networking disease, was spreading.

"There's a theoretical possibility that patients in areas where we hadn't currently shown the ticks to be established could have Lyme disease," (Harvey Artsob, director of zoonotic diseases and special pathogens at the *National Microbiology Laboratory* in Winnipeg).

There were predictions of worse to come: …"we expect, as our climate continues to warm… we're going to have an extension of our Lyme problem," (Dr. Kevin Forward, the head of microbiology for Capital Health in Halifax, Nova Scotia).

The Disease/Infectious News in England published the following report on May 29th, 2005:

"Lyme disease, an infection carried by ticks, causes a rash and stiffness in the joints and, if left unchecked, can affect the central nervous system, causing tingling in hands and feet, or facial palsy. In the worst cases the disease can also affect the heart, liver and spleen and even lead to encephalitis, which can kill. Depression and chronic fatigue grip many patients and ruin their lives."

The journal reported that in Scotland the number of sufferers went up 35 percent between 2003 and 2004.

"In England and Wales there were 97 cases 10 years ago and 320 in 2003. Specialists believe that the true incidence could run into the thousands because people, doctors and vets do not know much about it and do not seek treatment."

"Anyone who goes to the countryside is at risk for infection and the disease can also be picked up in parkland where there are deer. City-dwellers who visit parks such as Richmond, Bushy or Victoria are at the same risk as a stalker in the Highlands or a visitor to a stately home …it is also widespread in the United States, Germany, Hungary and the Netherlands and also exists on every other continent. Between 10 and 20 percent of British victims are thought to have contracted the disease abroad.

Many believe that it should be made a notifiable disease in England and Wales, as it is in Scotland. British military personnel and their families already have to notify their medical service if they get it.

Many people may possibly be carrying the antibody after a tick bite years ago, but show no symptoms, and in those cases the full-blown disease can be triggered by another illness or severe stress. Lyme disease can be difficult to identify as it mimics other diseases and the symptoms are not identical for every sufferer."

The skeptics may insist that there is no such thing as chronic Lyme disease, but hard evidence that there is just keeps piling up. Marjorie Tietjen, Director for Lyme concerns in the Common Cause Medical Research Foundation, is among many Lyme sufferers who challenge the 'Quackwatch' skeptics:

"Regarding my own case," she said, " I was not diagnosed until eight years into the disease. I was told I had Chronic Fatigue Syndrome, which, of course, has no cure – only symptomatic treatments. This late diagnosis resulted in tertiary or late stage Lyme disease with much brain and nervous system involvement. At this point I was very grateful to have found a doctor who has had success in treating many chronic Lyme patients. I know from first hand experience that chronic active Lyme is real and that the longer one goes without treatment, the more difficult the microbe is to eradicate. I was headed for total disability but thanks to the few brave doctors out there who treat chronic Lyme, I am now leading an almost normal life. It's an obvious example of cause and effect. Patients are sick with a chronic illness, they are treated with appropriate doses of antibiotics, for the needed length of time and, so, most people significantly improve. I really don't see why there should be a controversy, unless, of course, the controversy is related to politics and profits."

Conspiracy?

Added to the controversial nature of the medical implications of Lyme, there is also a growing suspicion of conspiracy surrounding this disease.

Much has been written about the U.S. government's so-called 'secret' experiments on Lyme as a bioweapon carried out on Plum Island. It is true that Plum Island (off Long Island and in close proximity to Lyme, CT) was , in fact, a 'classified' US Government animal disease research laboratory, between 1952 and 2004. In February 2004, Planet News broadcast the following on a book about Plum Island.

1975 The Lyme Connection (Michael Christopher Carroll . Publ. William Morrow Feb 2004)

From the 'PLANET NEWS' broadcast:

Plum Island is a small island off the coast of Long Island, NY. The author was interviewed this morning on the Today Show. A biological time bomb? This new book tells the story of the U.S. government's secret Plum Island germ laboratory and claims it's a ticking biological time bomb none of us can safely ignore. It sounds like the script from a science fiction movie. Dozens of deadly and rare biological diseases, housed on a bucolic island just a stone's throw from some of the wealthiest homes in America, with a history of contagious outbreaks, poor security, official denials, and perhaps most frightening of all, a potential terrorist target. Unfortunately, it's not science fiction. According to "Lab 257," a 2004 book by Michael Carroll, it's exactly what's going on just hours from New York City at the Plum Island Animal Disease Center in Long Island, New York."

Carroll discusses the book on Today. If you want a well documented book on the strange and somewhat bizarre business of the USDA and the military working on diseases like Lyme, West Nile virus, Foot and Mouth disease, etc., you should read this book which is listed on Amazon.com!

Patricia Doyle has also written on the connection between the USDA use of Plum Island for biowarfare research and the pro-Nazi German scientist Erich Traub who was employed as a tick researcher on Plum island. This is part of her research into Plum Island's history even before it became the USDA's top security animal research center. The history goes back to 'operation paperclip' (the secret file on Traub's and other pro-Nazi scientists' background and employment in the U.S) and to what she calls PROVEN tick research on Plum Island dating back to the 1950s. (See: Rense.com 'Plum Island, Lyme disease and operation Paperclip- a Deadly triangle' by Patricia Doyle Ph.D)

Whether there is some truth to the 'conspiracy theory' about Lyme disease and its virulence is somehow connected with biowarfare research; the fact is that the laboratory description of the Lyme bacterium appears to include a quite remarkable number of extraordinary attributes all pointing to its alarmingly suitable character as a bioweapon:

Distinguishing Characteristics of the bacterium *Borrelia burgdorfer* (Bb)

Internal Flagella
Glycoprotein Coat
DNA Net Arrangement
Bleb Formation
Prolonged Replication Time
Cellular Invasion Ability
Cyst Formation
Destruction of B-Cells
Camouflage as B-Cell
Internal Antigenic Proteins
Surface Antigen Transformation
Spiral Shape

From 'Biochemistry of Lyme Disease: Borrelia burgdorferi' (by professor Robert W Bradford and Henry W. Allen)

(See : The Townsend Letter February/ March 2006)

In the light of what's now known about this terrible disease, one thing is indisputably clear. We need to find a way to combat it or at least to contain it. The Lyme bacterium is capable of causing a worldwide disaster on the scale of the Black Death of 14th century Europe, which was also caused by the bite of a tiny insect carrying a deadly bacterium (*Yersina Pestis*). The Black Death took millions of lives in Europe. In England approximately 40% of the entire population died of Bubonic plague, the most famous form of the Black Death. England wasn't finally free of it until the 17th century. No one likes scare-mongering, but it makes no sense to dismiss the possibility of a similar plague in our own time. The global spread of AIDS should be enough to make that possibility clear. Containment is essential when we're faced with a global killer we don't understand as yet.

A clinical study of Lyme disease, its structure and method of attack as well as of its symptoms, makes good sense. It is our only option if we are to find a treatment that is successful other than in the earliest stages of the disease. Once Lyme takes hold, the accepted treatment with antibiotics becomes inadequate. There's the question of co-infection, disguised or 'copy-cat' symptoms and other stratagems used by this elusive bacterium.

4

THE WAR AGAINST LYME:

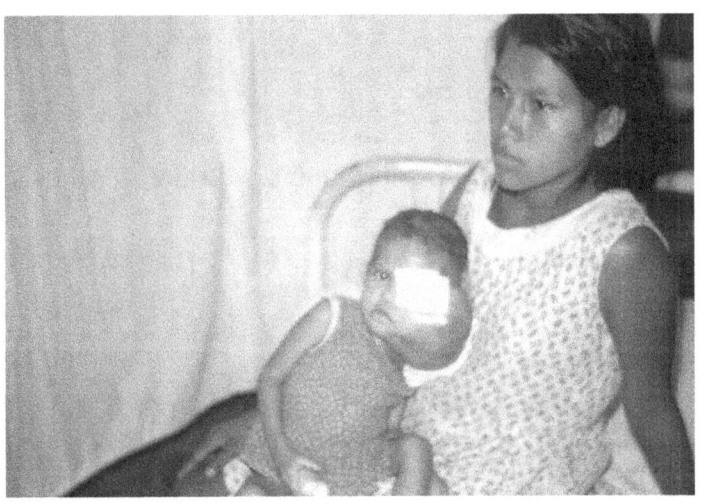

Baby with large Parotid land tumor which was inoperable. This child lived in the jungle of Peru on the bank of the Amazon river.

✿ ✿ ✿

There are many examples of government apathy or worse when it comes to public awareness of Lyme disease. Skepticism is alive and well. The Canadian Lyme

Association, for example, fears that the disease may reach epidemic proportions before public information is made mandatory. Here is an extract from a recent letter sent by the Association to the Canadian Health Authorities:

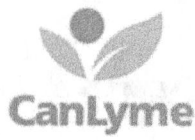 **Canadian Lyme Disease Foundation**
2495 Reece Rd. Westbank, BC Canada
V4T 1N1 www.canlyme.org
Ph:250-768-0978 Fax:250-768-0946

March 21, 2007
Hon. Tony Clement
Minister's Office - Health Canada
Brooke Claxton Building, Tunney's Pasture
Postal Locator: 0906C
Ottawa, Ontario, Canada
K1A 0K9

Hon. Vic Toews
President of the Treasury Board
Treasury Board of Canada Secretariat
L'Esplanade Laurier, 9th Floor, East Tower
140 O'Connor Street,
Ottawa, Ontario, Canada
K1A 0R5

Dear Hon. Clement and Hon. Toews,

Attached is a copy of a letter sent from the Board of Directors of the Canadian Lyme Disease Foundation to the Public Health Agency of Canada (PHAC) regarding the shameful and misleading way Canadians with Lyme disease and their representatives from our organization have been treated by government employees under the umbrella of the Public Health Agency of Canada…

A National Meeting on Lyme Disease funded by taxpayer dollars took place in March 2006. We were invited to attend and to provide expert speakers which we did. A representative for our organization participated on the planning committee for this national meeting. Recommendations at the closing of the conference were that committees were to be formed to arrive at consensus for the best practices guidelines. We were to be represented on those committees.

As it turns out this was a massive deception, and money from the public purse was expended to carry out the deception as outlined in our attached letter. The recently formed Canadian Public Health Laboratory Network (CPHLN) for which PHAC provides a secretariat had already formed a committee to set Lyme disease policy without stakeholder involvement. We only found out by accident that guidelines had already been created outside of our promised participation…

There is alarming and solid evidence of Lyme disease in the brain tissue of up to 70% of people diagnosed with Alzheimer disease, in the bowel linings of those with Crohn's disease, and in the blood of a high percentage of those diagnosed with Multiple Sclerosis, Chronic Fatigue Syndrome, Fibromyalgia and many other disease processes. Some of this substantiating research has been published in well-respected medical journals by our board members. John Scott, a published scientist, lyme disease victim, and head of the Lyme Disease Association of Ontario for 16 years has shown without any doubt in his research that Lyme disease is transplanted at random throughout Canada by our friendly migratory birds. Dr. Judith Miklossy's published research, which has been validated by other global researchers has clearly linked Alzheimer's to Lyme disease.

If Lyme disease is as rare as we are led to believe by these civil servants, how does one reconcile the well documented high incidence of Lyme being found in these diseases that are collectively destroying the lives of so many Canadians while draining our health care budgets? Why do these civil servants feel they do not have to address this issue in an open forum? Lyme disease will only continue to spread in coming years. This is a very serious matter now and in the future for the public health of Canadians…

The concern of the Canadian Lyme Foundation is mirrored by a general concern among many members of the medical profession that there is too little interest being shown by our governments in educating the public about the threat of Lyme.

The following web sites are among many that express that concern:

http://www.openeyepictures.com/index.html
http://www.lymenet.org/
http://www.lymediseaseassociation.org/
http://www.columbia-lyme.org/index.html

A war is being waged against Lyme disease but also against the lack of concern which seems to be based on an element of denial within our government health organisations. A major obstacle is the difficulty of diagnosis. Traditionally, the surest way of finding out if a patient has a disease is by laboratory testing. But this is precisely where the present confusion and controversy have their origin. Today there still no 100% accurate diagnostic test for Lyme disease. Most labs that test for Lyme infection have a poor sensitivity and a dependability rate of approximately 50–60%. This is why the diagnosis of Lyme disease is a *clinical* Diagnosis. Laboratory testing only helps to confirm the presence of the disease and cannot be depended on to make the diagnosis!

In other words, *a thorough history of the patient's symptoms is the most important factor in making a diagnosis of Lyme infection!*

One of the most accurate Labs that test for Lyme infection is IGeneX in Palo Alto, California. The sensitivity of their tests approaches 90–95%. Their tests are PCR, ELISA and Western Blot. They also test for co-infections from other tick diseases.

As regards lab testing for Lyme, the following scenario is often like this – a patient sees their doctor for what may be Lyme's symptoms and has his/her blood tested for the infection. The results return to the physician who tells the patient that since the test is negative he/she probably does not have Lyme disease! This does a terrible disservice to the patient involved since a negative result should never contradict the clinical symptoms of the disease!

I have talked to many a patient who has had just that same experience with their local medical doctor. And the reason is simple: their local MDs have not been properly educated regarding the enormous variety of symptoms to which Lyme patients are subjected. You really cannot blame the busy doctor who, though well educated in general medicine, has so little medical school information on the Lyme disease characteristics; and in spite of even speciality training, misdiagnose on a regular basis cases of Lyme disease.

Just recently I came across a case of a 30+ year-old daughter of a good friend of mine who developed some of the classic neurological symptoms of chronic Lyme disease. She saw two specialists in the field of neurology who both agreed that she had Multiple Sclerosis and began treatment (which never cures!) using injectable medicine "to help the patient manage the disease" with the pronouncement that "there was no cure and the symptoms will probably get worse in time." What a discouraging shock to the patient this pronouncement must have caused!

She later checked with what I call a LLMD (Lyme Literate MD) who had her tested with the San Diego IGeneX lab. She tested "very positive" and was immediately started on antibiotic therapy which is standard treatment today!

By the way, at the beginning of my writing this book, only one State in the U.S that had not reported a case of

Lyme disease – Montana. So if you don't live in Montana or plan to move away from Montana you need to read these stories for your own understanding of a growing menace to the population of not only the U.S but to the entire world.

There is a growing list of books about Lyme Disease written from the patient's point of view. Here are some titles:

<u>The Widening Circle</u> (Paula Murray, copyright 1996 Reed Business Information, Inc.)

Murray, an artist and mother of four from Lyme, Conn., (!!) tells of her tenacious struggle to convince doctors that she and her family were indeed sick, and not hypochondriacs, after they were afflicted by a mysterious illness. In the 1960s, Lyme disease, the tick-borne infection then unheard of, began its invasion of the Murray family. Frustrating rounds with doctors, referrals to specialists and batteries of medication became the family modality, documented in records of the puzzling ailments kept by Murray. In 1971, Murray, vilified as a "doctor-chaser," began her own systematic research, seeking out investigative medical personnel and sharing stories with fellow sufferers. A lonely journey that attracted media attention also attracted the attention of the medical community to the unusual cluster of cases in Lyme. In this exhaustive report, Murray has established a model by which <u>doctors must listen to their patients.</u>

<u>Confronting Lyme Disease: What Patient stories teach us</u>
Karen P. Yerges and Rita L. Stanley (Paperback, the Mitre's touch Gallery 2005)

There are several documented case histories in this book that will give you some in-depth understanding of the way in which Lyme disease treats its victims.

A 12 year-year old girl, Lauren, who had just finished sixth grade in May 1999 and had Summer plans already made. She was planning on going back to her home town in Wisconsin to see some of her old friends and that was when she was bitten by a tick and developed Lyme disease. It is a poignant story well worth the time to read.

The story becomes really interesting and complicated when she goes to the Emergency room with her symptoms of early Lyme infection and is referred to a Pediatrician who decided that the bites on the patient's leg were probably spider bites and not tick bites. The young girl (Loren) was given Amoxicillin and told to recheck with her Oregon physician in 3-4 weeks. In the meantime, Loren was suffering from all sorts of joint pains, backache, lack of energy etc. So when she saw her physician in Oregon, he renewed her Amoxicillin for another 5 weeks. The situation only becomes worse and…you must read the rest of the story. This might happen to your child or to you!

In another story, a professor at McGill University in Canada becomes a Victim of Lyme and finds that she must struggle with her physicians as well as with her insurance company (over disability insurance) while trying to keep her job even though she is reduced to being a wheelchair patient. Everyone, including physicians, who reads this story (it began in 2000 and is still unfolding), will empathize with the professor.

The following articles and e-mail letters, drawn from my own correspondence, may be of interest to the Lyme patient and his/her physician. Names have been changed to protect the identity of the people involved.

Kate's Story:

Since 1988 I've had Lyme disease. Like so many others, it took a long time to be properly diagnosed. I'd been told I had MS, but I never believed that. When we found out it was Lyme disease, we were hopeful that I could rid my body of the infection. In 1997, my health deteriorated drastically. The Lyme had infected my brain and I could no longer take care of myself. My husband has been my caregiver and has also researched every treatment imaginable for Lyme disease. He took me for 90 hyperbaric oxygen treatments (which did help, but was not a cure). I received blood chelation, which was also helpful, but not a cure. Intravenous injections of antibiotics and anti-protozoans were tried for years. Many other treatment regimens were tried, all helpful but without curing the disease. I tried to eat healthy foods and took recommended vitamins and supplements, but I seemed to be fighting a losing battle. Then my husband heard about the Rife light machines. He talked to our sons-in-law (both engineers) and decided that there was some merit in this new treatment (method

?). But we couldn't find any machines on the market. In desperation, he had a machine built and for 17 months I have been using the machine weekly. The quality of my life has improved dramatically. I have horrible Herxheimer's and they are difficult to endure sometimes, but once the toxins are eliminated I experience a feeling of tremendous improvement. I had prayed for the Lord to lead us to a cure and I believe that the machine is it. I wanted to share my story with you in hopes that you will research this for yourself. It has saved my life when we thought there was little hope for wellness.

Kate

Sharna's story:

'Sharna', a patient and friend, wrote to me when I was preparing to write this book. Her story was absolutely astonishing, and my correspondence with her is therefore set out here in some detail. It took the form of a question and answer dialogue between doctor and patient.

Dear Sharna,

Whatever works for you – I will be glad to have your story so that others might have a glimpse of what it is to be a Lyme patient and perhaps become more educated about this serious infectious disease. I understand your thinking process has been somewhat "changed"? or just "slowed up".

I understand completely! I have been through the same thing. So please feel comfortable in answering the following 10 questions:

1. Question: How old were you when you found that you had Lyme disease? And what was the year?

I was 32 years old. The year was 2005.

2. Question: How did you find out that it was specifically Lyme infection? What tests were done?

I saw Dr. W_____. He had me send a blood sample to IgeneX Labs. The test came back positive. Dr. W_____ told me the results. Other doctors that I have seen saw it as M.S. and not Lyme disease. I had additional CSF(cerebral spinal fluid) Lyme tests from the above University hospital were performed in December of 2005. I can scan and email the results if you would like. I read some of those results. It appears that some of those tests were positive. They made some kind of claim that the tests were not FDA approved or something like that, so it could not be determined if I had Lyme or not.

3 Question: What was your experience with the medical practitioners who saw you? Give details if possible.

Answer: First I went to a local Immediate Care clinic and told them about my headaches and blurred vision. The PA there referred me to Dr. X____ who is an Ophthalmologist. She dropped the ball on me and did nothing but took my money and put glasses on me that didn't help the problem at all. She never referred me to anyone. I told her about all of the headaches and vision problems. That was October 2004. I then went to Dr. Y____ at the _____ walk-in medical clinic in _____ with right thigh numbness. That was some time in February, 2005. He ordered an MRI immediately and the results were lesions found. He then referred me to Dr. Z____ who is a Neurologist and Dr.__A_____ who is an Ophthalmologist. Dr. A_____ confirmed Dr. __Y's_____ suspicion of MS. Dr. Z___ wanted to put me on MS drugs. I took Copaxone for 30 days. I couldn't do it any longer due to serious site reactions from the needles and medication. We are talking cantaloupe sized bruising and swelling. I am allergic to surgical steel and many other metals. Sticking a needle into me every day probably caused some of it. Dr. A____ did the regular eye exams and nothing more. I saw Dr. Z_____ continuously throughout 2005. I then went to_____ MS Center for a second opinion. They just confirmed the data I supplied— the diagnosis of MS. That was in October of 2005. I stopped working September of 2005. I was then referred by Dr. A____ to the Ophthalmology Clinic at a well known University in California. The neuro- ophthalmologist, Dr. B____, admitted me to _____ Medical Center for a week of steroids via IV. He said I was legally blind and that is why I needed to be admitted—to keep things from getting worse. After 8 hours of testing.I finally came to this conclusion: That was positively the worst week I've had in my life. I truly felt like a lab rat. The confusion of student residents, inconsistencies, lack of communication, and stressed out residents, attendants and nurses was more than I could take. A resident doctor performed a lumbar puncture then they sent me for an MRI–the same hour no less. Before that I was allowed to get up to go to the restroom instead of using a bed pan. BIG MISTAKE. After that my head was in so much pain they finally gave me morphine but only after they gave me codeine which I told them I was allergic to. I vomited constantly causing the lumbar puncture to continue to leak. They then gave me a blood patch. That seemed to help. Saturday morning, the fifth day at the medical center, they tried to give me another IV course of steroids. They had trouble with my veins since day one. I told them they had one chance to find a vein. If they couldn't find it then I was walking out. They couldn't get a vein and I yelled at them and told them to discharge me and not to touch me again. I think that might have been the steroids talking. I left Saturday morning. They then gave me a prescription for Prednisone. They did not tell me that I had to take the tapering off dosages and what would happen if I didn't take it. By the time I got home, my head was swimming still. I felt like I was on a small boat out in the middle of the ocean with very large waves. I saw Dr. Z_____ the next Monday. He saw that I was taking Prednisone. They didn't help. I felt completely crazy. I stopped taking the Prednisone on Tuesday. I then went into adrenal failure. I was flat on my back for weeks. The entire attempt to mask my problem didn't work one bit. I do have better balance today—7 months later. However, I have severe bladder incontinence that I didn't have 7 months ago. My poor eyesight is still the same. All of the doctors that I saw except for Dr. W_____ have denied that I have Lyme. I tried the hyperbaric chamber 6 times. While I was in the chamber, I had to take Ativan because of extreme sweating and anxiety. The last three treatments that I went through caused my eyesight to deteriorate tremendously. I was even sitting relaxed on a guerney (spelling?). It got better after I was out of the chamber for a while.

4. Question: Tell me about yourself and your environment before you received the IgeneX positive lab report on your Lyme infection?

Answer: I was adopted and have never met my biological parents. My adopted parents moved to Northern CA when I about 2 years old. I was always outside in the dirt playing with cats or mud pies. Sometime between 2 and 5 years old I was bitten by a tick at the nape of the neck. I didn't even know it was there. My mom pulled it off, killed it and threw it into the toilet. I also contracted ringworm on the chest from holding cats on my chest. We lived on _____ Rd at the time. We then moved to _____ Rd where I was constantly outside and playing with either a dog or a horse. I rode horses through the local area brush for years. I never noticed a tick biting me during that time. I did find them crawling on me from time to time. I was around flies and mosquitoes constantly and got bitten a lot. I rode horses in Paradise, Durham, Chico, Oroville, Grass Valley, Sacramento, Pleasant Grove, and Vacaville. I was fine until the Summer of 2004. I noticed my eyesight becoming blurred when I would walk around or when I got stressed out. I've always been weight challenged, but

I always felt fine and had energy to burn. I did have a gallbladder removal procedure in 2000.

5. Question: What treatment did you start at the beginning, and what are you doing at present to combat the problem?

Answer: Dr. W_____ put me on Zithromax and then Doxycycline. He stopped that and started Minocycline after a couple of weeks. I stopped taking that medication when I quit the hyperbaric treatment. The antibiotics did not help my already crippled digestive tract. I started taking Copaxone injections for 1 month in May of 2005. I stopped that. I was told by Dr. _____ that I needed to be on some kind of MS drug. I have refused everything. I have been doing pretty well until the heat hit. I drink a lot of carrot juice, water, and make good foods. I buy nothing out of a bag or box. I don't drink milk or eat anything from an animal. I get a lot of sleep. To keep my mental status healthy, I drive myself to feed and spend time with my horse at 5 a.m. every morning. My eyesight is at its best at that time of morning—right when I wake up. I need to keep from getting bored. I can't go take a walk. My legs buckle if I try to walk much. It just isn't safe for me to try to walk down the road. During the day I exercise by running in place and doing r Yoga-type moves. I do this until I become limp and then sit and wait until I can get on with my day. This is repeated a few times per day.

6. Question: Your parents' reactions to the diagnosis?

Answer: I honestly don't remember their exact actions. My mom drove me to work for a while and fed my horse. She was very helpful. They were saddened by the whole thing. I know that. When I had to quit a great job that saddened them even more.

7. Question: Any other family members with the problem of Lyme infection?

Answer: I don't know. No other family members have the same symptoms that I have. I don't know about my biological parents.

8. Question: Present program to get well? Activity? Antibiotics? Alternative treatments?

Answer: Just the daily routine of eating well, attempting to exercise. I try to schedule anything that my eyes have to see in the morning, since my vision gets worse as the day progresses.

9. Question: A list of symptoms as the disease progressed?

Where do I start? I'm most likely leaving something out.

Left side weakness in the arm and leg. Right arm and leg numbness especially in the bottom of the right foot. Vision loss, bladder incontinency at times. At first I had horrible headaches constantly. I then became incontinent of both bowel and bladder at my work place. I also got horrendous acid reflux. I thought an elephant was sitting on my chest at times. I still have that today. If I eat lots of raw vegetables, I get pain from stomach acid. My digestive system does not work like it used to. I can go 4 or 5 days with out a bowel movement. Then I will go with no problem. I don't get impacted. Dr. W_____ says my large intestine isn't working right. My keyboard typing ability has definitely been hindered. In 2003, I typed 87 wpm. That is one of the reasons I was hired at_____. Now I am lucky if I can type 35 wpm. Another problem is heat. If the temperature is more than 65 degrees in my environment, my vision immediately deteriorates. Everything becomes foggy and darkens. At times I ask my husband if there are clouds outside when there isn't one anywhere. I have become moderately color blind. My right eye is worse than my left eye. I am completely color blind when my eyesight gets poor. My balance is not as good as it used to be. If I stand with my feet together and close my eyes, I will fall forward. I can't stand in the shower because of the heat either. I used to have twitching in my legs and sharp, stabbing pains at the back of my neck in 2005. Those have not returned for a while.

10. Question: How does all of this affect your school, recreation, and general health index?

Answer: I can't see well enough to take classes. I can't work. I can't remember well or concentrate like I used to. I have to write lists for everything. I have to make a mental list of what to do when doing the simplest tasks such as taking a shower. I can't drive during the day when the sun is out. My depth perception has been limited. If someone doesn't tell me that I will be walking down steps, I'll fall down them. I get incredibly painful headaches above and behind my right eye approximately once per month. I can't lie flat on my back without getting nauseated. I can't be independent like I used to be. My husband has to drive me to all appointments and shopping excursions. When we go shopping, we can't dilly dally. We make a list and go as fast as we can. I get weak and sometimes have to sit on the floor in the middle of the store. Luckily, Winco has a refrigerated beer locker. I go in there to try to get my strength and eyesight back. I buy most necessities online because my husband doesn't want to run around and shop on his days off of work; therefore, I pay more for items and have less money. I can't do what I need to do in obtaining supplies for my horse. I have to pay extra to have things delivered. When having conversations with someone, I have to ask what the topic was. When I get a train of thought, I have to finish it. If I am interrupted, I will forget the entire thought. I used to be great at multi-tasking. That is another reason that I was hired at _____. I am unable to multi-task anymore. Even if the phone rings, I lose my entire thought process and forget what I was working on. Almost everything I have learned from college education in the last three years is pretty much gone. I also lose my eyesight when I eat. If I haven't sufficiently answered this question, please let me know if you would like me to elaborate on anything. My ups and downs have mainly been depression. My husband, though he meant well, tried to physically keep me from driving. He didn't understand that I can see well enough in the morning to drive. I have to really focus on the road and watch for things in the road such as people, cars, and animals. He learned to trust me. That was a bit of a power struggle. I miss the money and benefits that I had from working. I am now on Medi-cal with a $1,200 co-pay. That doesn't do me a lot of good when it comes to the smaller appointments. That will just keep me from having to pay $65,000 for a hospital visit. I mainly miss not being able to jump in my truck and go shopping. I miss not being able to stand in the kitchen to cook. I miss not being able to see the TV screen after I've been doing something or eating. I miss not being able to search the Internet like I used to do. I miss not being normal. I finally told all the doctors that I have been working with that I want nothing to do with the medical community. If they haven't figured out what causes MS by now…why are they not willing to think outside the box and consider Lyme as a cause….if they unable to think outside the box, I refuse to be a "lab rat" any longer.

Hi, I don't know if I mentioned these ups and downs. Ups–I get to stay home all day.

Downs–depression. The University docs wanted to put me on Prozac for being depressed. I replied with "If you were in my condition you would be depressed too.!" I'd rather feel my depression than mask it and not feel anything. Zombieism doesn't sound exciting to me. I am depressed for a reason. Since I know why, I can deal with it the way I want to."

Since all of this, I've also told doctors that I am the only one who really knows me. That's why I opted out of any further medications. I know if there is a side effect, I will get it--100% guaranteed. The MS drug Avonex may cause suicidal tendencies, liver problems, and the list goes on. NO THANKS!

As you might gather, I'm a little angry at my disease and the people who claim to be able to help me.

Anyway, I'll stop my ranting. I've stopped talking to anyone about it. If I do talk to someone I start crying uncontrollably. That's a bit embarrassing, so I don't talk about it anymore. On the bright side, it hasn't killed me yet.

Typing all of this and the answers to the questions has actually helped me quite a lot. I was able to type it without bawling my eyes out.

Thanks ☺

(notice how the dam broke when she discussed her symptoms and the way she was treated by doctors on her case)

Amy Tan's story

Amy Tan is a writer. Upon its publication in 1989, Tan's book, The Joy Luck Club won enthusiastic reviews and was (for eight months!) on the New York Times best-seller list. Paperback rights sold for $1.23 million.

The book has been translated in 17 languages, including Chinese. Her subsequent novel, <u>The Kitchen God's Wife</u> (1991) confirmed her reputation and enjoyed excellent sales. Since then Amy Tan has published two books for children, <u>The Moon Lady</u> and <u>The Chinese Siamese Cat</u> and two novels <u>The Hundred Secret Senses</u> (1995) and <u>The Bonesetter's Daughter</u> (2001). <u>The Opposite of Fate:</u> A 'Book of Musings', appeared in 2003.

This extract is taken from 'Amy Tan on Lyme Disease' (www.amy tan/lyme.net)

"I have late-stage neuroborreliosis. I have had this disease since 1999.

My case is in many ways typical. Like many, I had little awareness of Lyme disease, for I did not live in what was considered the tick-infested hotbeds on the East Coast. I am a Californian -that's where I file my taxes- and I live among the hills of San Francisco with its tick-free, concrete sidewalks. For a good long while it did not seem significant that I also have a home in New York , that I weekend in the country, and my main form of exercise is hiking. In addition to trekking in the woodlands of Mendocino, Sonoma , and Santa Cruz counties in California , I have also sojourned to leafy spots in Connecticut and upstate New York . I once loved to sit in the tall grass next to the river, and lean my back against a shady oak tree.

I passed off my early symptoms -a stiff neck, insomnia, a constant headache, and a bad back followed by a frozen shoulder- as the unpleasant aftermath of too much airplane travel. I was often tired and jittery, but that, I reasoned, was the consequence of an active and exciting life. Who was I to complain? I had a wonderful life, a great husband, lovely homes, a successful career. I was rarely sick and went to the doctor only for my annual checkup. Even when I came down with the fever, aches and pains of the 'flu' earlier in the summer, I had managed to beat it back without developing any of the respiratory sequelae. What a great immune system I had!

When my feet grew tingly and then numb, I mentioned to my doctor that I had had an unusual rash earlier that year. It had begun with a tiny black dot that I guessed might have been a pinprick-sized blood blister. It grew more rounded as it filled, and then I either scratched it out or it fell out on its own, leaving a tiny pit and a growing red rash, which, curiously, did not itch, but lasted a month. Because that rash seemed so unusual, as did my neuropathy, I wondered aloud whether they were related. My doctor said no.

Like many chronic Lyme disease patients, as my symptoms mounted and a scattering of tests proved positive for an array of seemingly disparate conditions, I was referred to specialist after specialist, until I eventually had consulted ten and had taken countless lab tests .....Hallucinations began, what I now realize were likely simple partial seizures, the result of lesions on my brain. I saw people walking into my room, two girls jumping rope, numbers spinning on an odometer, a fat poodle hanging from the ceiling. I also had strange episodes in which I behaved strangely but had no recollection of what

I had done as reported to me by others. I apparently rang people up at midnight and talked in a wispy voice. I had flung laundry around the living room. My husband said I acted at times as if I were in a trance, eyes wide open but unresponsive to his and a friend's questions. I now had nightly nightmares and acted them out, punching at lamps or my husband, and once landing on my head in a dive toward my dream assailant....

....I turned to the Internet, which is where doctors believe patients catch terminal illnesses, that is, whatever disease they see described before them on the terminal. And there I saw that an ELISA was also used to screen for Lyme disease. Further reading led me to see that all my symptoms could easily fall under the multi-systemic umbrella of borreliosis. Further sleuthing gave me the name of a Lyme specialist, someone my other physicians acknowledged was 'a good doctor.'

My Lyme specialist considered the history of my rash, the summertime flu, the migrating aches and neuropathy, the insomnia and fatigue. He thought 15 lesions in my brain were significant in light of my neurological symptoms. He saw on previous tests that I had some interesting changes in my immune system. He ordered a complete battery of tests from IGeneX, a lab specializing in tick-borne illnesses, to check for not only Lyme disease, but its common co-infections. Two weeks later, I learned I was positive for Lyme on the Western Blot. My doctor told me that the test only confirmed what he already knew....

....Like many late-stage neurological Lyme patients, it took a while for symptoms to begin to lift. A day after starting antibiotic treatment, I became feverish and ill with the classic Jarisch-Herxheimer reaction. A month later, the joint and muscle pain eased up somewhat. Two months, and some of the fog finally lifted, and I frantically wrote for long days, fearful that the curtain would come down again. After six months, I had no muscle stiffness or joint pain remaining. Today, I can once again write fiction, speak at conferences, and walk in my neighborhood alone and without anxiety and panic. I've been under treatment now for over a year. I consider myself 85% improved from where I was a year ago. I still have what I call memory black holes when I am tired, and I have neuropathy in my feet, which at times becomes too painful for me to walk more than a block. I know that my late diagnosis means I am in this for years, perhaps even for life. But at least I have my mind back."

As a patient, I have joined a club of people with a stigmatized disease that many doctors do not want to treat. While I have been lucky enough to find a doctor who is willing to provide open-ended treatment -and I have the means to pay for it- many of my fellow Lyme patients have gone without appropriate care. As a consequence, they have lost their health, their jobs, their homes, their marriages, and even their lives.

I now know the greatest harm borrelia has caused. It is ignorance. Lyme disease is more prevalent than most people think. It is more difficult to diagnose than most doctors think. It requires more research before we know how it can be adequately treated, and one day, cured.

In the meantime, my advice to friends and family is to be aware and be informed. Realize that Lyme disease has been reported in every state except Montana. The CDC estimates the actual numbers of those infected each year is at least tenfold of what is documented as cases. Some Lyme specialists believe the numbers are even higher than that.

And if you are bitten by a tick and suspect you have been infected, go see a Lyme-literate physician. Get treated early and adequately. Don't wait, as I did, and let a treatable disease turn into a chronic one."

Of course Amy Tan is a fine writer, a creative artist with words; so we might wonder if perhaps she has 'overdramatised' her experiences. But she has not exaggerated her symptoms nor her dreadful experience at the hands of the medical practitioners whom she consulted. She decided to consult a psychiatrist for the first time in nearly 20 years; the doctor in turn suggested she also get a complete medical workup.

Finally, after comparing what she knew with what other patients reported on the ILADS Web site (www.ilads.org), Tan discovered Rafael Stricker, a Lyme specialist in San Francisco .

Stricker says Tan's 'clinical symptoms and history were very suggestive: striking psychiatric problems and hallucinations, which you can see with Lyme disease.'

He tested her with a Western Blot, and had it analyzed by IGeneX.

Stricker says Tan has tested positively on the Western Blot five times in a row. Among the 16 antigen bands that IGeneX identifies, her tests 'have been pretty uniform,' with positives for seven or eight bands each time. She has consistently tested positive for two of the three bands the CDC considers accurate indicators of Lyme, he says. He considers her diagnosis conclusive.

As she concludes in an essay from her upcoming book 'The Opposite of Fate' : 'I am in this for the long haul, with treatment that will likely last for years. I won't feel safe until the scan of my brain and blood tests on my immune system return to normal, until the Western Blot is negative for Lyme disease, and my myriad symptoms are gone. . . . By having Lyme disease, I have automatically been drawn into the medical schism over both its diagnosis and treatment.'

'I now know what is the greatest damage that *Borrelia* has caused: It is ignorance."

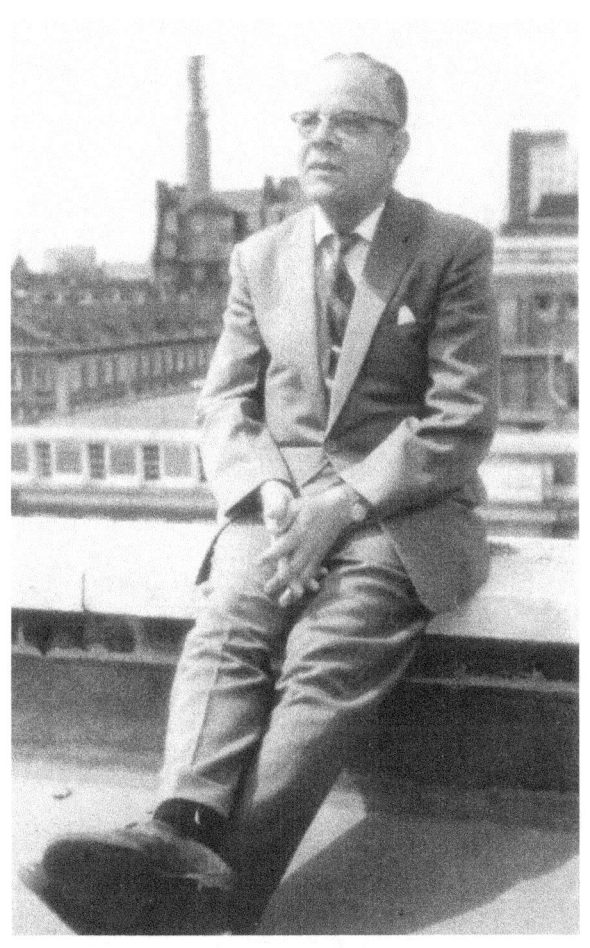

The author's father in his mid 70's

5

A MEDICAL PUZZLE SOLVED

❊ ❊ ❊

(My father's sudden, 'inexplicable illness' after 100 years of healthy life)

My father was a retired pharmacist, an avid scrabble player and a well-liked person in the community. He spent the last 25 years of his long life with my youngest sister's family in Manitoba, Canada.

His physical health was outstanding. He neither drank nor smoked, loved the physical exercise of swimming and walking and had lived an abstemious and admirable life. At 99, he was still able to mow the lawn and would walk at least a mile or more every day.

That was about the time he began to show symptoms of an illness that seemed utterly foreign to him. Dad was almost a stranger to illness because of his healthy life-style. Even a common cold was a rare occurrence.

Now he began to develop a maddening itch all over his body, that no medicine seemed able to relieve. He had constant itching over his entire scalp which became progressively worse to involve the entire upper torso. He was seen by a succession of 5 physicians and an acupuncturist to no avail. The itching which showed as a red rash on his chest continued unabated until a dermatologist started him on high doses of Prednisone (a cortisone product). He seemed to be getting better after 2 months of medication which was gradually reduced over a couple of months.

When the medicine was finally stopped, he developed hallucinations which were sometimes so real that he would be mortally afraid for his life. In one incident, he saw tiny crying babies floating into his room at my sister's house. He also saw strange people standing outside and trying to enter the house forcibly. He also developed a cardiac arrhythmia (termed PAT) - a rapid heart beat that made him feel very weak and faint. This was treated with anti-arrhythmia medicines which worked most of the time. He finally stopped taking the medicine and did just fine for the next year. A year later, he had to be taken to the local hospital by ambulance for what appeared to be a light stroke which occurred at the breakfast table.

The findings at the hospital were paroxysmal tachycardia which was terminated by electro-conversion (using the emergency electric chest paddles). In the meantime, Dad was starting to hallucinate and was very angry and shouting at the staff to find out why he was there at the emergency room. From here, it all starts going downhill over a period of 9 months which moved Dad from the medical intensive care to the Psychiatric ward, to the placement unit, and finally to a very nice nursing facility run by the Salvation

Army. I was there with him in May and also in August/
September. My two sisters and I saw him twice daily while
he was still in the hospital and later when he was transferred
to the nursing home. The drugs in the hospital were not
doing much more than making Dad a total "vegetable" –
unable to feed himself and go to the toilet without help.
His balance became very unstable and he hallucinated
every 3-4 days. Below is a letter I wrote to the physicians
who attended my Dad:

9/17/2006

To: Dr._____

Re: William Alfred Gilkes

Dear Dr._____

I am taking this opportunity to congratulate you and your
colleagues on your new hospital facility in _____ and
to let you know my appreciation for the high standard of
care given by the nursing staff in spite of the chronic short-
staffing of hospitals both in the U.S. and Canada.

As a physician with a California license I am interested
in my father's case regarding his unusual symptoms which
have changed almost daily and are very baffling due to the
fact that he has no specific diagnosis which can be treated
with a reasonable expectation of a final cure. This patient is
100 years old and normally would be considered old enough
to be having a form of dementia or some type of psychotic
problem.

Fortunately, I have been present in _____ staying
with my two sisters who have spent many hours on a daily
basis working with their father – feeding, cleaning dentures,

helping to walk with a walker and generally engaging him in conversation to keep his mind active. My daily observations of the above patient since <u>August 15th, 2006</u> to the present date have been very enlightening. After many hours of consulting my sisters' diary notes re: my father's health condition for the past year, I noted the following facts:

1. William Alfred Gilkes (WAG) was able to mow the lawn outside of his previous residence without any untoward side effects up to age 99. He also would walk up to a mile or two almost daily.

2. WAG played the word game known as Scrabble and would easily win even when playing some of the best local Scrabble players! He was a "master scrabble player" His vocabulary has always been excellent and his speech (English) impeccably accurate. His past profession was a pharmacist and he has lived in California, England, and Canada for the past 22 years with my sister Marsha who has been a resident of Brandon for approximately 31 years.

3. While living in California he lived both in the city and the country areas and stayed many years in Lyme endemic areas of the State.

4. Approximately 3 years ago, WAG developed what was diagnosed as PAT (paroxysmal atrial tachycardia) and was treated a number of times via the Emergency Room of the local hospital in Brandon. He was placed on a calcium blocker and that seemed to prevent the PAT most of the time. About a year later WAG discontinued the calcium blocker. He was completely

asymptomatic until just recently when he was hospitalized for an apparent "stroke", which was not verified by MRI or other tests.

5. About a year ago he complained of pruritis with what appeared to be an atypical case of Erythema migrans involving his chest and back areas. This erythema was treated by one of the 5 physicians who have seen WAG and who prescribed oral Prednisone "step down dosage"and topical hydrocortison for approximately 2 months. This seemed to calm the itching and the erythema until it was finally discontinued; whereupon the rash flared up again with increased pruritis which was relieved by cold compresses on a temporary basis. At present WAG has little or no pruritis, however, his skin in those areas has not returned to its original color.

6. During late November 2005 WAG developed some "visual type hallucinations" e.g. "rain falling before his eyes, muddy waters around on the floor, and other objects including people who were doing strange things inside the home. Some of these apparitions were so horrific that he became extremely agitated and actually felt that "demons" were going to eat him and kill him!

7. Since his latest hospitalization, WAG has experienced some minor hallucinations in spite of medicine which he is taking on a daily basis. Yet, he becomes almost 99% rational with good memory for recent and past events. This mental situation

changes almost on a daily basis and is interspersed with periods of <u>total fatigue</u> and almost the inability to carry on any kind of verbal communication.

8. I have personally witnessed his ability to walk with a walker one day and the next he is so fatigued that he sleeps most of the day. He does have <u>all night insomnia</u> which is unusual for him. This insomnia has been progressive for a number of months both at home and in the hospital. Any drugs for sleep make him a "zombie". After his Propanalol was reduced (in recent weeks in hospital) to 10 mg daily his mental alertness improved and his pulse increased from 50–64 per minute since the change...Within the last 3-4 weeks I have personally taken his pulse and noted it to be between 48 and 64. In the last week, it has been 60 or below during the evening when I usually accompany my two sisters who feed him. His motor skill for self feeding varies from day to day and some days he is able to feed himself without any help!

9. Within the last year WAG has complained of visual "blurring" and does have a past history of bilateral lens replacement. Apparently an optician in Brandon said WAG had "macular degeneration" Yet WAG can tell the time on a ladies wrist watch held upside down at approximately 3-4 feet away. The past 2 days have been amazingly different in that WAG has apparently recovered to usual mental "self" and thinks clearly and has a good memory for both present and past events! The moment he mentions seeing "rain falling before

his eyes" we know by experience it is heralding another episode of a few days of mental confusion and some hallucinations. This fortunately does not last for more than a couple of days.

10. With the subtle combination of –:

    a.   Erythema Migrans type rash

    b.   Total fatigue – recurring and lasting all day.

    c.   "Blurry vision". He keeps his eyes closed most of the time because as he states: "it makes my eyes feel more comfortable". Apparently, he is having a light sensitivity problem

    d.   Cardiac arrhythmias – intermittent.

    e.   Increasing insomnia.

    f.   Hallucinations, with Paranoia and occasional semi-violent behavior (<u>rare</u>)

    g.   Has lived for a number of years in Lyme endemic areas.

    h.   Has one son with diagnosed chronic Lyme disease and who lives in an endemic area for Lyme disease.

    i.   The development of various food allergies which have occurred within the last year. Apparently his reaction to certain foods spawns itching symptoms involving most of his skin surface.

    j.   Days of clear thinking and apparently normal behavior which is spectacular.

    k.   Chronic constipation over the past 1-2 years.

After "connecting the dots", I suspect that dad may have been suffering from mild to significant cerebral inflammation secondary to chronic latent Lyme infection of the brain. This turn of events may have been encouraged by Prednisone used for the pruritis which is no longer a problem.

My main concern for my father is not to increase his life span but rather to see that he is as comfortable as possible during the last days of his stay on this earth.

After reading this somewhat long "epistle", I am hoping you will be able to talk to me after you digest the material enclosed. My telephone numbers are included at the end of this letter.

Please find enclosed a number of items which may be of interest to you and your colleagues, since the increasing problem of Lyme infection especially in the chronic stages is now the most prevalent tick borne infectious disease in North America and has made major inroads in England and Europe.

At present, I am working on a book regarding this incredible "masquerader" spirochetal disease and hope to publish it by early 2007.

I will be available to talk to you or anyone in the medical field regarding the above items and would welcome the opportunity. I will be in Brandon until September 19th, 2006. I also plan to be back in Brandon sometime in the late Fall of the year.

Thank you for considering the above possibilities and wishing you and the hospital staff the best of success as you continue supporting a very modern and beautiful institution.

Yours respectfully,
Gordon A. Gilkes MD., MPH.

Note:

9/17/2006

Personal follow up of patient by patient's son Gordon A. Gilkes MD.,MPH. records that:

- Patient Alfred Gilkes has had a pulse of 60 and below for over 3 weeks (my personal evaluation of this patient). <u>Pulse was taken in the late afternoon</u> at supper time.
- On 16th of Sept. 2006 both hands and feet were edematous and cold to touch with some signs of poor circulation.
- Patient has been chronically <u>constipated</u> since admission to the hospital.
- Patient has been having <u>hallucinations </u>while in the hospital since May '06.
- Patient has had some <u>minimal tardive dyskinesia</u> problems during different times I have observed during the past few weeks.
- Patient has had recurring <u>serious insomnia</u> lasting all night for the past few weeks.
- Also <u>fatigue, lethargy and vivid dreams</u> have been noted.

Suggestions:
- Stop all Beta-blockers or reduce dosage to one every 2nd day.
- Stop Loxapine on a trial basis to see if some of the serious symptoms clear up. Or decrease significantly.

- Since being in hospital, patient was given Cipro for approx. 10 days for what was said to be a urinary infection (first time he has ever had one!} he responded mentally and was considerably improved from a psych. standpoint. Perhaps he may respond to a trial of Doxycycline 100 mg BID or Cipro BID for a couple of weeks. This would be on a trial basis of course. <u>Patient is allergic to Penicillin products</u>.

- To highlight how sensitive this patient is to medications – when he was staying with me in California a few years ago, he was treated by a Gastro-Enterologist for H. pylori stomach ulcers. He was given as part of the Rx. Prevacid (H-2 blocker). WAG lost his ability to speak within 48 hours and even though could write legibly and have all his motor abilities untouched, he was unable to utter one understandable word!.

- In fact he was unable to vocalize any words!

  On removal of the offending medicine, he regained his speech ability within 24 hours. The medicine was again given to him on a trial basis and sure enough, he again lost his speech at which time the specialist discontinued the Prevacid! The specialist had never seen a reaction like this in his entire career! Incidently, the PDR (physician's desk reference) does mention that occasional "rare neurological "effects may be noted!

Thank you for your attention to the above. You may call me anytime at the following telephones after 20th Sept.'06.

_____ home phone.

_____ cell phone

Before the above date you may reach me at _____ or

_____

Yours truly,
Gordon A. Gilkes MD. MPH.

....
****
....

This was not sent in the letter above since it an addendum to Dad's illness. After the doctor stopped the antibiotics (Cipro) which Dad was given for a mild pneumonia Dad did very well indeed and was very lucid and able to converse and even feed himself for at least 3 weeks after the discontinuance of the antibiotics. Then without warning, he began declining again and was having more trouble swallowing food or liquids. This became chronic over the next month or two until he finally lost his ability to swallow normally. In the meantime he was losing weight rapidly and not wanting to do much more than sleep and doze all day long with occasional intervals of awareness. Dad then started refusing all oral liquids and solids. An IV was started and he was obviously not happy with that even though his speech was limited. He finally passed away on the 22nd January 2007, 6 months away from his 101st birthday...

There was no diagnosis made except "<u>inflammatory areas of the brain</u>" causing patients demise. It took the pathology department in Winnipeg 3-4 months for the report to be made! The general autopsy did not show any physical problems so the family requested an examination of the brain in the main pathology lab stationed in Winnipeg.)By that time, all spirochetes would have been destroyed and invisible to the microscopic exam!). As far as I know, the only tick-borne disease test done was an Elisa test as per the CDC standards. This was negative!

6

A REPORT FROM THE
FRONT LINE:

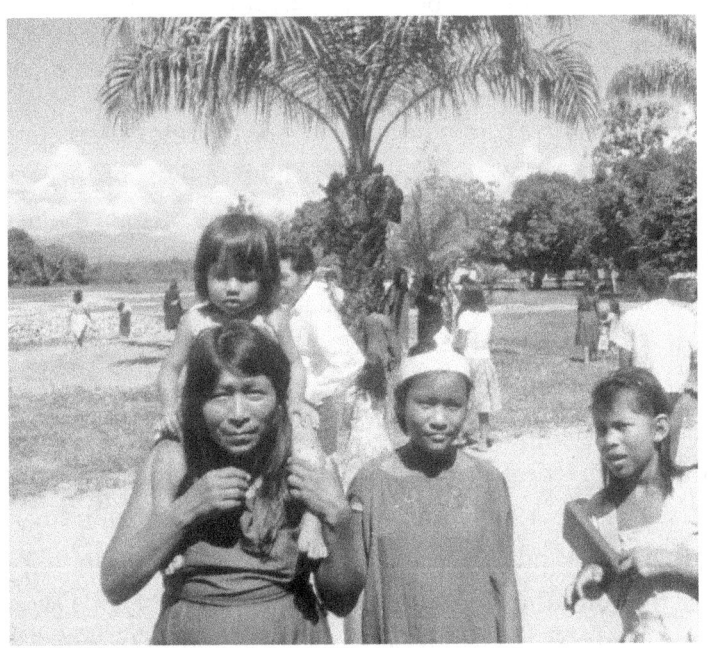

Natives living in the Amazon jungle of Peru

❧ ❧ ❧

First, let me fill in some professional and biographical background to this report. My wife and I were both born and brought up in South America where we lived until young adulthood. We met in the U.S.A. as university students during our medical/nursing studies there. My own graduation from medical school was followed by internship and a period of wide experience in Emergency medicine and surgery. My wife graduated as a nurse with special interests in nutrition. She has co-authored with our daughter (also a nurse and graduate in Public Health) and published a bilingual cookbook – with both English and Spanish recipes.

After our two children were born, we decided to go back, as a family, to South America to spend some time there and to offer our services to those who were less fortunate than we were. We also needed the challenge of something different, perhaps more demanding. By doing so, we would be following the spirit of that sentence in the Hippocratic oath : "I will remember that I remain a member of society, with special obligations to <u>all</u> my fellow human beings". At the same time I felt that I could learn something more about the practical, 'hands-on' aspect of the profession I had chosen. So, in 1967 I volunteered to go overseas with my wife and two children (8 and 4 years old) to live in Iquitos, Peru to run a mission hospital sponsored by the 7th Day Adventist church. We left our home in California to travel to the ancient land of the Incas. Our final destination was a remote jungle outpost in Iquitos near the headwaters of the Amazon river and the heart of the rainforests of Peru.

A humid blast of jungle air hit us in the face as we stepped off the little plane that had flown us over the Cordilleras. After our years in California, we had almost forgotten how different and 'in your face' the climate is in an equatorial setting. We had stopped overnight in Mexico City and then arrived the next day in Lima, Peru where we spent a few days with the directors of the Adventist mission program in South America.

Running a jungle hospital and clinic in the Amazon Basin, working with the Peace Corps and raising two bright, active and healthy children, we were kept very busy.

We quickly became acclimatized and I started seeing patients almost immediately, since the previous doctor was already preparing to leave after his tour of service. The realization soon dawned on me that I was about to become director, medical assistant, chief surgeon and outpatient physician of the outpost all rolled into one. The year of intensive surgical skills training I had received in central California would now be put to the acid test. The nature and variety of the medical/surgical cases I was about to encounter would add enormously to my practical experience of medicine and surgery. Here, for example, I would see my first case of leprosy. I attended to a patient with the typical epitrochlear lymphadenopathy (enlarged lymph nodes around the elbow area) and skin areas of the back that had lost feeling. I knew that I would also have to make unusually tough decisions.

One such case was a pregnant 50 year old mother of five with Miliary tuberculosis. The successful treatment of the disease would almost certainly entail the termination of her 3 month pregnancy. But attempting to saving the fetus would almost certainly mean her death. I opted to treat the disease and she recovered fully and was able to return to her jungle home to look after her other 5 children, though the foetus was lost via a surgical abortion.

That was the most difficult decision I have ever had to make in my entire medical career...

I remember draining an epidural hematoma (a large blood clot inside the skull pressing against the outer covering of the brain) in a 17 year old male who had fallen out of a tree and was admitted to the local military hospital (his father was a soldier connected with the local military contingent) for observation and then sent home since he was awake and ate a meal. He became unconscious for the second time when we saw him in our makeshift emergency room. This consisted of a single table adjacent to the surgical room with its bare concrete floor, an air conditioner protruding from the wall of the room on the other side. The hematoma was successfully drained after opening the skull using a sterilized drill bit on an antiquainted brace and bit instrument. We used a "gigli saw to raise the cranial skull bone above the hematoma to visualize the blood clot over the damaged brain area.

One particularly bizarre case was that of a young girl who, while swimming near the bank of the Amazon (in the nude, as the children there usually did) experienced great vaginal pain and bleeding because of a small sharp-finned fish which had swum up into her vaginal canal. I'd never seen anything like this before and was fortunately able to remove the creature and save the girl from more serious damage. I later learned that this fish and its alarming and dangerous predilection was well-known to the native population. They called it "el carnero" (the butcher).

Once, a very young boy had been attacked by a bull as he attempted to cross an open field on his way to school. He was gored through the mouth by the bull's horn which pierced the roof of his mouth causing severe damage to the sinus area. He recovered from surgery without any major after effects.

In this environment one had to learn to be innovative as well as decisive in surgical procedures. One case that I shall never forget was the gunshot injury of an escaped prisoner. He had been shot through the right side of his chest and was brought in by the same police who had shot him. The man had no pulse, wasn't breathing, but was still warm to the touch. My new assistant and I virtually brought him back to life by suctioning off the blood that had settled in the right lung and had not clotted (thanks to a special enzyme produced by lung tissue) into some vacuum bottles containing a chemical to keep the blood from clotting. We placed an intravenous line in his arm in spite of the difficulty of finding the collapsed vein, and auto-transfused his own blood from the lung cavity back into his body via the IV line. We inserted a chest tube to drain off any remaining fluid over a period of approximately 10 days. The man fully recovered. In fact his recovery was so remarkable that when I enquired how the patient was doing, now back in prison in solitary confinement, I was told he had escaped again!

When my stint of service was over, my family and I returned to California where we finally found our "Shangri-La", a beautiful home in the gentle, wooded slopes of the Oroville hills. After working with two Emergency departments of hospitals in the area, I established my own practice : an Urgent and Routine Medical Clinic (URMC). I had learned a great deal about the practice of medicine in rudimentary and far from ideal conditions. It had been an exciting as well as sobering experience. My missionary medical work made me even more appreciative of the crucial role physicians often play in a community.. The URMC would be an expression of what for me was now both a vocation and an avocation.

For ten years, between 1985 and 1995, I managed the URMC, located in Paradise, California, as Physician–in–Charge. During this period my family and I lived in our beautiful home just 20 miles from the clinic and enjoyed country living with pine trees and oaks all around us in a setting we thought was almost a paradise. I enjoyed walking in our 5 acres of land which gave us enough room to grow lots of fruit trees. The lower end of our property was mainly brush and weeds which attracted deer that sometimes jumped the fence to nibble the grass. They also liked nibbling the rose plants my wife lovingly cared for. I would run down the hill at the back of our house with our Labrador dog running ahead to chase the deer. I spent many hours working away with a brush-cutter to clear the weeds. It was a great way to get exercise especially after a busy day at the clinic in town. Of course I often got a few scratches and insect bites in spite of wearing long sleeves and long trousers. I preferred to do this rather than use insect repellent. This was our little, nature-friendly "heaven on earth" and everyone who came to visit us immediately fell in love with our "haven in the hills."

After a while I again felt the need for a challenge, another change of perspective and routine. Eventually I decided to leave the URMC life and in 1995 joined the State of California Dept. of Corrections as a rank and file physician. Every week I would drive the 100 miles to work at a prison in Susanville, CA. I would stay in the city during the week and come home on the weekends. After four years of working for the State of California my family and I decided to move temporarily to the Susanville area. By this time I had been appointed Chief Medical Officer.

I have always enjoyed good health and always felt energetic. After a year in the new job, however, I began having difficulty seeing clearly while driving at night especially when the white lines on the roads were poorly defined or missing. At first I simply wrote this off to the ageing process. I was looking forward to retirement anyway. But this was just the beginning of an even bigger change: a change for the worse.

In 2001 I retired from the CDC (California Dept. of Corrections).

Retirement at last! We moved back to our hill-side country home which we had rented in the interim. I felt great, and started working again in our idyllic, hillside Nature garden. I was soon cutting weeds, walking, doing all the activities I enjoyed and living the outdoor life I loved.

Then in 2004 I decided to do something about a painful tooth. I visited my favorite dentist's office. The tooth had been hurting on and off for at least a year, and because the X-rays did not show up any problem, I put up with the pain until, finally, I had to have the tooth pulled. My dentist found a huge eroded area of bone in the lower jaw where the tooth had rested. This was a surprise to us both and necessitated a total cleanup of the jaw bone cavity using a bone graft to fill the empty space left where the bone had been eroded.

Within days I developed a virulent "flu infection" which resisted all my efforts. I used the tried and true household remedies I often gave my patients : lots of fluids, bed rest, herbs, fruit etc., but this 'flu episode lasted for about 4 weeks. I became so weak that I could hardly get out of bed! This I told myself, was not normal! I wondered whether the surgery on my jaw that might not have caused an infection even though I had no fever. My dentist had me come in for another X-ray. The X-ray showed normal healing and absolutely no sign of infection.

Finally, as I became more mobile, I went again to see my dentist who still could not find any sign of infection even though I felt terribly sick! I was very depressed at not being able to make a diagnosis since the blood tests that my doctor had run showed that everything was normal. This was a medical puzzle until my dentist asked me if I had ever thought it might be Lyme infection. That was the first time I heard the term 'Lyme infection' mentioned by any of my health care providers.

As I recovered slowly from the "flu syndrome", I decided to do a search on the internet. I typed in the words "Lyme disease". The flood of information that I released was simply astonishing. I was now determined to research every nook and cranny of the subject of Lyme disease. In pulling my tooth, a dentist had opened my eyes !

Now I began to understand why I had "arthritis" in my fingers, wrists, knees and spine. Now I knew that my "blurry" vision was not necessarily due to "early cataracts" but might have been the result of retinal damage caused by an infection. I'd had German measles in my late 30s which affected my perception of colours, but not of my clear vision. Time took care of the colour problem, but the recent "blurry". eye problem and incredible light sensitivity continued unabated. My eye surgeon didn't share my diagnosis of Lyme disease. He then referred me to a retinal specialist The specialist could not explain the damage to the retina.

Then I remembered that my thumbs had developed severe tendonitis even before I had the eye problem. I had found that I could not straighten them without experiencing pain which became worse as time passed. My thumbs remained involuntarily curled inwards. I thought back to my stint as prison doctor. Could it have been caused by the constant trauma of opening heavy prison doors with very large door keys? The prison physicians carried their own door keys to open clinic doors etc!

For the first time I began to connect the dots. Some of my health problems had seemed 'unreasonable', since I had always been in good health. And now I also remembered how, when out walking with my wife, I would suddenly feel sharp, stabbing, needle-like pains for a second or two in my right and sometimes my left thigh. My knees would occasionally be sore on some days but perfectly normal on other days. It was beginning to make sense at last! My symptoms might perhaps be all connected with the infection.

Finally, I came across the Canadian Lyme Foundation web page (www.canlyme.com) and checked out all the possible symptoms listed.

I had 47 of the 75 listed symptoms!

So with my own potential diagnosis in hand, I presented all the facts to a Lyme Literate physician(an MD. who has some background in the area of Lyme disease and is willing to listen to my related symptoms) in my area. He agreed with my diagnosis and shared with me some of his patients' experiences. He also gave me a prescription for antibiotics which I dutifully started taking. He suggested that I take them for one month and recheck with him to decide how much longer I should be on the antibiotics since my case was 'obviously chronic' Lyme infection. The Lyme test he had me take had come back <u>negative</u>, yet he felt sure I had Lyme disease symptomology!

I trusted his judgement but after a week on the antibiotic (Doxycyline 100 mg twice daily), I developed severe itching in the rectal area and even with appropriate medication there was no relief. I also felt dreadfully ill because of the antibiotics. I have never tolerated antibiotics very well, and was always very careful about how I prescribed them for others in my previous practice. So I broke a standard medical rule. I quit taking the antibiotics without telling my doctor! I did more research on the Internet and talked to others who have had similar responses to antibiotics. Today, I suspect that I was having a Herxheimer reaction (Herxheimer's reaction which is the result of toxins liberated in the body due to "kill off" of the bacteria. That might also explain why my reaction to the antibiotic was so severe.

I tried another approach: colloidal silver 250 ppm (parts per million – Yikes!) one half teaspoon daily orally. That didn't last very long either. You might want to do your own research (scientific) re:the danger of this practice!). Yet, I have met and talked to several folk who used colloidal silver preparations with excellent results not only for Lyme symptoms but also for rapid relief of sore throats and even eye infections!! This is something I am still unable to understand!! Today, physicians still use topical silver preparations for burns, and other skin lesions with good results – but orally? Never! Well I didn't plan on "turning blue" from Argyria caused by ingestion of colloidal silver products! Those cases are usually rare and the dosage is usually very high and the concentration of the product is suspect.

Meanwhile I was sleeping 3 or 4 times during the day but never really felt rested. My brain was fuzzy and I was having difficulty with all but the simplest of words. That really frustrated me! I felt nauseous, especially at bedtime, and my body temperature fluctuated between internal chills in the day and sweating at night.

My vision wasn't getting any better either. Then a breakthrough came. I started Hyperbaric Oxygen therapy which was recommended for neurological problems including MS, Lyme, Post CVA(stroke), cerebral palsy, and a number of other conditions like the "bends" due to a diver surfacing too quickly after a deep dive in the water. The increased oxygen pressure in the hyperbaric chamber allows oxygen to enter the body even through the skin as well as the lungs. This increased oxygen to the body's tissues promotes healing of wounds and has saved many a patient's extremity from being amputated due to non-healing lesions secondary to diabetes etc. For example, one of my family members avoided a foot amputation by the use of this technique. So I opted to go that route and had a month of 4 days-a- week Hyperbaric chamber treatments.

I was given almost immediate relief. I could go home after treatment and walk up the hill near our home and actually race ahead of my wife (who is an avid walker) on the home stretch after walking for at least 2 miles! I was feeling so much better because the extra oxygenation of my body was giving me much more energy and drive. In the meantime I started an interesting-looking course on Real Estate. I knew that I had to keep my brain working to counteract the feeling of 'mental laziness'. That , I now know, is one of the most insidious symptoms of Lyme disease.

During the last week of Hyperbaric Oxygen therapy I noticed a little more "blurring" of my vision than usual, and, in checking up on this effect, I realized that high oxygen pressure could cause problems of circulation in the retina, especially if there is already inflammation of that area. So, though it gave me a huge boost, I had to dispense with hyperbaric Oxygen therapy just when I felt that I was getting well again. Since then, I have met other folk who have done the same therapy and feel they have been successfully cured of Lyme symptoms.

I tried to regain something of the energy and drive I had felt before by working in the garden, but I still did not have that vitality. I also developed pains in every muscle and joint that was involved in the outdoor activity. Perhaps that's one reason why so many Lyme disease patients tend to be overweight. They probably avoid exercise because it makes them hurt too much afterwards. I now use a 4 foot wide trampoline to do gentle exercises to keep my lower limbs and extremities active and supple, and I walk as much as my body will let me.

2004 passed quietly, without incident. I did some Real Estate transactions and got my feet wet in this booming market. I was kept busy planning all sorts of ways to buy and sell Real Estate successfully. Yet there was always that lingering "tiredness" and visual challenges that dogged my footsteps. I was working 6 days a week (half days only) and enjoying it even though I had to be careful to avoid any extra stress (tell that one to any real estate agent!).

2005 came far too quickly. I was able to complete a number of Real Estate transactions even though I did not feel like my normal self. To others I seemed well enough, but I knew that my body's batteries were low. There is a familiar question often aimed at those suffering from Lyme disease: "How come you look so good but feel so bad ?" It may be well-meaning, but it can seem bitterly ironic to the Lyme victim.

Then came another breakthrough. I found out from my research that with the manufacture of 'wave therapy' machines that produce Photon Emissions via a Resonant Light source could possibly give me another weapon of attack against Lyme infection, a way of controlling pain symptoms and possibly reversing some of the damage done by the spirochetal attack. This machine is also tagged under the general term of "Rife" machine technology. It is not FDA approved in the US, and has been registered by the Canadian authorities under the category of "Tens" equipment for pain control. I believe, at present, it is only approved for use on animals. A number of vetinarians use this with good results in their practice of animal medicine. What really started my thinking was an article in a Bio-Engineering Journal (which I have lost) that showed how seriously depressed patients could be totally cured by passing electrical currents through the back of the nape of the neck via the vagus nerve. Here is an Internet article which is pertinent to the above Rx. http://149.142.238.229/k30/reading/Vagus_Nerve_Stimulation_Art.pdf

But first let me tell you about the method one of my dentist acquaintences told me he used to fight and defeat the Lyme infection. It's a remarkable, if somewhat unusual story. He said that he'd never had such a terrible backache in his life – enough pain to keep him from working with patients for some time. With many other symptoms he was diagnosed with Lyme disease and opted for his own home-style Hyperthermia therapy (heat treatment to selectively kill bacteria) since the spirochete that causes Lyme disease is susceptible to increased body core temperature.

He rigged up a bathtub with hot water at a temperature of 105+ degrees and soaked in it daily for approximately one hour for over a month. He claims he no longer has any symptoms of Lyme! He did admit, however, that the treatments were like "going to hell and back" daily. He was the second person who has told me the same story. Unfortunately I have very sensitive skin and I am sure that I could not handle that hot water treatment for any length of time. This method is sometimes used in cancer treatment, and oddly enough, it is precisely how medical practitioners treated patients with the spirochete of Syphilis many, many years ago. I must say, though, that I don't recommend this treatment without some trained personnel in constant attendance!!

There are two main types of photoelectric Wave Therapy machines: <u>Contact types</u> where the user has to make contact with the machine using hands or feet, and <u>Photon Emission Resonant Light</u> type machines. The latter is not as popular because of their higher cost, but very easy to use since the patient doesn't need to be in contact with the machine.

When I heard that there was a non-invasive method of immobilizing and finally killing the Lyme spirochete I was intrigued, since I needed something besides antibiotics and herbs. I wanted to get completely well without swallowing pills for years as many Lyme patients do. Even after downing many hundreds of capsules these patients often still have a lot of symptoms that just won't go away. This has been called "post-infection syndrome". Actually, in my opinion, it is a continuation of the infection which has not been totally defeated. This belief is still being investigated by various groups interested in defining some of these concepts.

So after extensive investigations and talking directly to Lyme patients who were using their Photon Emission Resonant Light machines I decided to purchase one even if I had to use my credit card and pay it off little by little. My maxim has always been that money spent for health is money well spent. Of course, this was another of my interesting "experiments".

I began using the machine which is pre-programmed with different 'banks' and frequencies that have been used by thousands of people who have reported good results attributed to certain frequencies As far as I know, there have been no reports of any problems from those users...

I started with the 'General Health' bank which ran frequencies from 10000 Hz to 20 Hz with each frequency lasting a few minutes. The machine did this automatically and had a special read-out attachment to let you know how far along you were in the approximately ½ – 2 hour treatment. After my first treatment was over, I awoke (the machine let me nap during the 1 ½ hour session) feeling refreshed and more energetic than usual. Even my aching muscles felt better! So the next day I tried bank #10 which is more specific for Lyme disease treatment. This went well until I remembered that if the treatment did in fact maim or kill some spirochetes I would probably have a Hx reaction (Jarish-Herxheimer reaction). And sure enough, within another 8 hours I started feeling like a truck had run over me! This went away after another approximately 6-8 hours had gone by. What an experience! Lately, those reactions have become less and less, and I am feeling more energetic as all symptoms are subsiding, but not completely gone. I can tell already that this technique will be a long term program with - I hope! – a gradual reduction of treatment days. It is basically a personal experiment that I don't recommend for anyone unless they are personally convinced it will help them based on their own research which includes contact with others who have used the machine. In this area we are all on uncharted ground.

I have heard the remark that since "there is no absolute proof that the machine works why use it." Yet we use so many devices e.g. various herbs, medicines, saunas, medications which make us feel lots better though we do not know exactly how they work. In the case of antibiotics, we have some knowledge of the actions of these but rarely ever consider the incredible side effects that are suffered by so many of us who use them. If you pick up the Physician's Desk Reference (PDR) and take any drug in that book as an example, you will find that the side effects are listed. If patients knew of these possible side effects, they would hesitate to take most drugs dispensed by the medical/pharmaceutical industry. You take a calculated risk when you swallow <u>any</u> pill whether prescribed by a doctor or a practitioner of herbal or 'natural' medicine. Most patients take more medicines than they really need. When I was running the URM Clinic in the 1990's I spent a large amount of my time helping patients reduce or eliminate medications that were doing them no good at all. Part of the problem was the patients' habit of 'doctor shopping'. They would collect pills from every doctor they saw and by the time I came in contact with them, they usually had a big paper bag full of medicines they didn't need. I think here it may be good to mention that although antibiotics have side effects – the side effects for many who tolerate them well are insignificant to the side effects and addictive nature of the many hard drugs used by some medical doctors to treat individual symptoms of Lyme disease. These range from steroids, to addictive and harsh narcotic pain killers to anti-psychotics which people in many cases must be carefully weaned from before commencing antibiotic therapy once a Lyme diagnosis is made

From my research, I have learned that the Lyme spirochete takes on various forms:

1. The typical corkscrew shape that allows it to bore into any tissue or organ at will. This is the most susceptible form as far as antibiotic treatment goes.
2. The L-shaped form which is less violent with tissues and is an intermediate form before becoming a cyst.

3. The cyst form which is the almost indestructible form that attaches itself to the deep tissues to protect itself from the onslaught of antibiotic therapy and other chemicals introduced into the body's environment. The cyst form usually coats itself in an almost impervious mucous covering which protects it from harm. [There is recently published research about the spirochete residing intracellularly in collagen making it an almost impossible target for antibiotics]

The cyst form becomes a spawning ground for future spirochetes because as it hibernates in the deep tissues of the body, forming tiny granules on its outside coating which later turn into new spirochetes. When the cyst decides that the environment will permit it to return to the spirochetal form (the active form) then the symptoms return with added strength. This exactly mirrors the behaviour of recent terrorist organizations, which are expert at playing hide and seek. Lyme disease spirochetes, the terrorist within our tissues, is even able to re-arrange its DNA/RNA format in order to fool the human immune system into thinking it is harmless! Now you know why this disease is so pervasive and persistent and why therapy needs to last for many months and even years. The 'war' against Lyme disease is going to be a long one.

The good news is that those who follow a reasonably healthy lifestyle seem to have less symptoms and resulting sequelae from Lyme infection than others who make little or no attempt to live healthfully.

There are 8 rules to health that spell NEWSTART. If more people followed them they would have stronger immune systems and be able to overcome diseases faster and with lasting results. Here are those simple rules -:

N = <u>Nutrition</u> with healthy foods, especially rich in vitamins and minerals. Lots fruit and vegetables and 'whole foods' which are not processed.

E = <u>Exercise</u> on a regular basis depending on age and physical condition.

W = <u>Water</u> taken internally : about 8 glasses daily.

S = <u>Sunshine</u> in moderation. Avoid sunburn through overexposure.

T = <u>Temperance</u> in all things.Avoid poisons like tobacco/alcohol etc.

A = <u>Air</u> As fresh and as clean as possible.

R = <u>Rest</u> Try to get enough sleep to improve your energy storage. For some, a short nap in the day works also.

T = <u>Trust</u> in Divine Power which can be a great healing influence.

Everyone is a unique individual, and no one treatment works the same way for all. This is a fact of life. In the case of Lyme disease, the patient has to <u>want</u> to learn as much as possible about his/her problem and sometimes has to use common sense and sometimes experimental evidence which can be gained in many ways. Physicians who are experienced and knowledgeable in identifying Lyme disease can be very helpful; but the patient must invariably take control over his/her own health and trust the physician as a general guide who should be willing to discuss possible treatment programs which must be tailored to the particular patient's situation.

A good physician will always listen very carefully to a patient's symptoms and will be aware of the various tried and tested techniques that may help.

So how am I doing at present?

Well, I'm still fighting off the Lyme intruder. Relief from my symptoms is sporadic but encouraging. And here I am, writing this book so that others can have an easier time figuring out the problem and not have to rely 100% on the medical profession to make a diagnosis. Waiting for a medical diagnosis can be fraught with delay and lack of first hand knowledge regarding the Lyme syndrome.

Today I can almost make a tentative diagnosis on the phone when someone calls me to find out if they could possibly have Lyme disease. How can that be possible? Simply because Lyme disease requires a clinical diagnosis and in the majority of cases, the symptoms are obvious (if you know what they are!) and all you have to do is connect the dots. Lab tests are confirmatory rather than diagnostic. They assist the health practitioner to be more confident of the diagnosis. I know this is a long term battle due to the incredible survival skills of the Lyme intruder, especially in its cyst form. So unless one is willing to persevere for a period of not less than 6–12 months and often much longer, there will not be a permanent cure.

I also understand that some doctors believe that you can cure the problem in 30 days or less with antibiotics. This is only possible if the infection is caught within 30 days or less after the tick bite. The problem is that the majority of patients are not diagnosed until many months to years after the start of the infection, and the majority don't even remember being bitten by a tick. The idea that chronic Lyme infections can be cured in 30-60 days is a false assumption which has been proven wrong over and over again. Unfortunately many Medical Boards believe in the "short term" idea; so much so, that they have actually threatened some of their physicians who use long term antibiotic therapy with the withdrawal of their licenses.

I have opted to use alternative methods to overcome my symptoms and hopefully be free from the disease without long term antibiotics. The reason is simple, and personal. Long term antibiotics will not work in my case because of my intolerance to most antibiotics. Yet, I will always keep an open mind and not be "fixed" on the above statement!

Even where there is no serious allergic reaction, long term antibiotic therapy can give many patients a host of side effects that are sometimes worse than the disease it is meant to eradicate. There is an increase in yeast infections and the overgrowth of other bacteria that normally do not have a chance to multiply thanks to the normal intestinal and body tissue defense mechanisms. Antibiotics kill all kinds of bacteria, not just the ones you are targeting.

So long-term courses of antibiotics can lower your immune system which is then unable to keep in check the many virus and bacterial invaders that we fight off on a daily basis. In this scenario, the patient should be taking well established pro-biotic products which enhance the intestinal flora and reduce the number of side effects.

On the other hand, I think it should be pointed out that tens of thousands of people are on long-term antibiotics on any given day in North America with very few side effects and side effects that are entirely manageable. I don't think we should imply that long-term antibiotics=problems, because in so very many cases it does not, and that is the only way many people manage this illness after trying all other methods. So there you have it! Both sides of the same coin! The pros and the cons of antibiotics.

Incidentally, I recently received a lab report from IGeneX which was positive for Babesia, a co-infection which is rarely a single infection. The lab report is simply a confirmation of the clinical diagnosis. The Babesia infection was not so obvious since it can mimic some of the Lyme symptoms. That makes it (using the language of modern warfare), an 'insurgent' force working alongside Lyme, the terrorist intruder. Incidentally, Babesia is rarely found by itself; it usually accompanies Lyme 98% of the time according to some estimates.

I hope that my story will also help to expand your own knowledge and understanding of this rapacious and persistent disease, and that physicians who read this book will discover some of the 'hidden' characteristics and details of Lyme disease from a fellow physician in the front line of the battle. My own fight against Lyme disease is not over: I now know that recognizing the enemy and understanding its strategies are essential prerequisites for success.

Meanwhile, the fight goes on.

PART TWO

THE LYME NETWORK;

7

TICK BORNE CO-INFECTIONS WITH LYME DISEASE

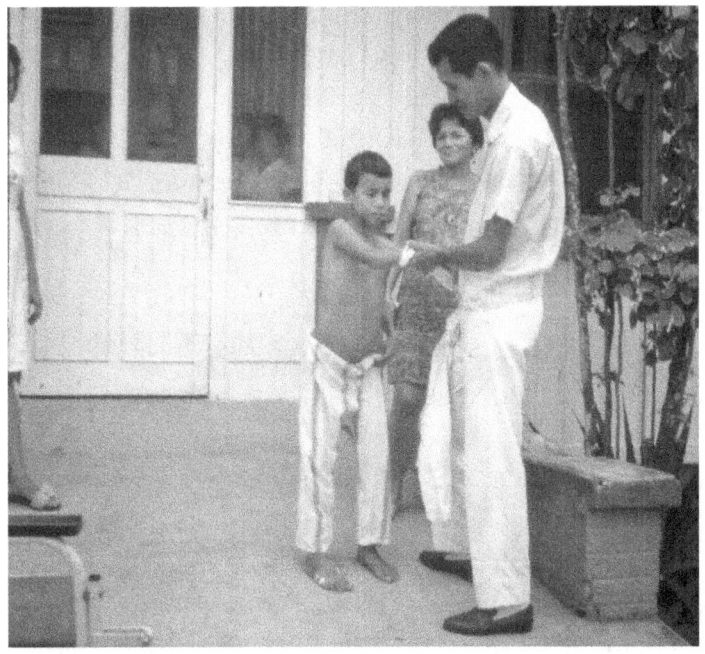

Jungle hospital in Iquitos, Peru. Patient with medical assisting doctor demonstrating a recovering case of Tetanus. This is not a tick borne disease but rather from an infection caused by a germ found in fecal contaminated wound from a sharp object.

❈ ❈ ❈

Lyme can be called the 'networking' disease. It has the ability to mimic but also to connect with other diseases, often using their presence to further its own advance. Here are some of the connections, or co-infections, as they are called. Needless to say, co-infections help to complicate the diagnosis and treatment of Lyme disease.

The following information comes from the <u>International Lyme and Associated Disease Society</u>

CO-INFECTONS with LYME:

Babesiosis, <u>Ehrlichiosis, Bartonella</u>. (also other tick-borne diseases – Tularemia, Tick Paralysis, Tick borne relapsing fever[1] and Rocky Mountain Spotted Fever)

<u>BABESIOSIS</u> (Piroplasmosis) (for critical research also read this: <u>Clinical Microbiology Reviews, July 2000, p. 451–469, Vol. 13, No. 3</u>)

GENERAL INFORMATION

Piroplasms are not bacteria; they are protozoans. Therefore, they will not be eradicated by any of the currently used Lyme treatment regimens. That's why co-infections are significant: if a Lyme patient has been extensively treated yet is still ill, suspect a co-infection.

See <u>Dual Infection Worsens Lyme Disease Symptoms</u> (www.Niaid.nih.gov/publications/dateline/0996/page3.htm)

Babesia infection is becoming more commonly recognized, especially in patients who already have Lyme Disease. It has been claimed that as many as 66% of Lyme patients show evidence of co-infection with Babesia. It has also been reported that Babesial infections can range in severity from mild, subclinical infection, to fulminant, potentially life-threatening illness. The more severe presentations are more likely to be seen in immunocompromised and elderly patients. Milder infections are often missed because the symptoms are incorrectly ascribed to Lyme. Babesial infections, even mild ones, may recrudesce and cause severe illness. This phenomenon has been reported to occur at any time, even up to several years after the initial infection. Furthermore, asymptomatic carriers pose risks to the blood supply as this infection has been reported to be passed on by blood transfusion, and to the unborn child from an infected mother as it can be transmitted in utero. Some quotes from the literature:

Krause, PJ. Spielman, A, Telford, SR et.al. Persistent parasitemia after acute Babesiosis N Engl J Med 1998. 339:160

"The clinical spectrum of human Babesiosis ranges from an apparently silent infection to a fulminant malaria-like disease."
"When left untreated, silent Babesial infection may persist for months to years."
"Silent infections, which occur in about a third of infected people, may recrudesce."

"Babesial infection may recrudesce after many months of asymptomatic parasitemia."

"Although parasites were initially detected microscopically in the blood of two of the untreated subjects, and all of the treated subjects, none could be found a week after the onset of illness."

"Persistent symptoms of Babesiosis accompanied persistent blood-borne Babesial DNA."

"The persistence of seroreactivity increasingly correlated with the persistence of Babesial DNA."

"In those with only subtle symptoms, Babesiosis often remains undiagnosed."

"Furthermore, physicians tend not to recognize Babesial infection in those who are co-infected with the agent of Lyme Disease, because Babesial symptoms tend to be ascribed to Lyme Disease."

"Physicians caring for patients with moderate to severe Lyme disease should consider obtaining diagnostic tests for Babesiosis and possibly other tick-borne pathogens... especially in patients experiencing "atypical Lyme disease" or patients in whom the response to antibiotic treatment is delayed or absent."

Krause, PJ, Telford, SR, Spielman, A, et.al. Concurrent Lyme disease and Babesiosis. JAMA 1996. 275 (21):1657

"Subjects with evidence of both infections reported a greater array of symptoms than those infected by the spirochete or piroplasm alone." "Co-infection generally results in more intense acute illness and a more prolonged convalescence than accompany either infection alone." "Spirochete DNA was evident more often and remained in the circulation longer in co-infected subjects than in those experiencing either infection alone." "Co-infection might also synergize spirochete-induced lesions in human joints, heart and nerves." "Babesial infections may impair human host defense mechanisms" "The possibility of concomitant Babesial infection should be considered when moderate to severe Lyme Disease has been diagnosed."

SYMPTOMS

In milder forms, symptoms may include a vague sense of imbalance without true vertigo, headache, mild encephalopathy, fatigue, sweats, air hunger and occasionally cough. When present as a co-infection with Lyme, initial symptoms of the illness are often more acute and severe. Suggestions of co-infection include the above symptoms, but the headaches are more severe, and encephalopathy is out of proportion to the other Borrelia symptoms. The fulminant presentations include high fevers, shaking chills and hemolysis, and can be fatal.

DIAGNOSTIC TESTS

Diagnostic tests are insensitive and problematic. There are at least thirteen Babesial forms found in ticks, yet we can currently only test for B. microti and WA-1 with our serologic and nuclear tests. Standard blood smears reportedly are reliable for only the first two weeks of infection, thus are not useful for diagnosing later infections and milder ones including carrier states where the germ load is too low to be detected. Krause, PJ, Telford, SR, Spielman, A, et al. Concurrent Lyme disease and Babesiosis. JAMA 1996. 275 (21):1660 "As is common in the case of Babesial infections, parasites frequently cannot be seen in blood films." Therefore, multiple diagnostic test methods are available and each have their own benefits and limitations and often several tests must be done. Be prepared to treat based on clinical presentation, even with negative tests.

SEROLOGY

Unlike Lyme, Babesia titers can reflect infection status. Thus, persistently positive titers or western blots suggest persistent infection.

PCR

This is more sensitive than smears for B. microti, but will not detect other species.

ENHANCED SMEAR

This utilizes buffy coat, prolonged scanning (up to three hours per sample!) and digital photography through custom-made microscopes. Although more sensitive than standard smears, infections can still be missed. The big advantage is that it will display multiple species, not just B. microti.

FLUORESCENT IN-SITU HYBRIDIZATION ASSAY (FISH)

This technique is also a form of blood smear. It is said to be 100-fold more sensitive than standard smears for B. microti, because instead of utilizing standard, ink-based stains, it uses a fluorescent-linked RNA probe and ultraviolet light. The Babesial organisms are then much easier to spot when the slides are scanned. The disadvantage is that currently only B. microti is detected.

TREATMENT

Treating Babesia infections had always been difficult, because the therapy that had been recommended until 1998 consisted of a combination of clindamycin plus quinine. Reports suggest that a more successful regimen is available to treat this infection. See http://aafp.org/afp/20010601/tips/3.html

Krause, PJ. Spielman, A, Telford, SR et.al.. Persistent parasitemia after acute Babesiosis N Engl J Med 1998. 339:162

"Of the treated subjects, almost half had symptoms that were consistent with reactions to quinine, including hearing loss, tinnitus, hypotension, and such gastrointestinal symptoms as anorexia, vomiting, and diarrhea." "Although treatment with clindamycin and quinine reduces the duration of parasitemia, infection may persist and recrudesce and side effects are common."

"Because of these dismal statistics, the current regimen of choice for Babesiosis is the combination of atovaquone plus azithromycin. This combination was initially studied in animals, and then applied to Humans with good success, because when atovaquone was used alone, resistance developed in 20% of cases, but reportedly did not occur when azithromycin was added. Fewer than 5% of patients have to halt treatment due to side effects, and the success rate is clearly better than that of clindamycin plus quinine. The duration of treatment with atovaquone plus azithromycin for Babesiosis varies depending on the degree of infection, duration of illness before diagnosis, the health and immune status of the patient, and whether the patient is co-infected with Borrelia burgdorferi. Typically, a three-week course is prescribed for acute cases, while chronic, longstanding infections with significant morbidity and co-infection will require several months of therapy. Relapses have occurred, and retreatment is occasionally needed. Problems during therapy include diarrhea, mild nausea, the expense of atovaquone (over $700.00 per bottle — enough for three weeks of treatment), and rarely, a temporary yellowish discoloration of the vision. Regular blood counts, liver panels and amylase levels are recommended during any prolonged course of therapy. Patients who are not cured with this regimen can be retreated but with higher doses, as this has proven effective in many of my patients."

"Artemesia (a non-prescription herb) may be added, but is not effective when used alone. Metronidazole can also be added to increase efficacy, but there is minimal clinical data on how much more effective this regimen is.

EHRLICHIOSIS (Human Granulocytic Ehrlichiosis)

GENERAL INFORMATION

While it is true that this illness can have a fulminant presentation, and may even become fatal if not treated, milder forms do exist, as does chronic low-grade infection, especially when other tick-borne organisms are present. The potential transmission of Ehrlichia during tick bites is the main reason why doxycycline is now the first choice in treating tick bites and early Lyme, before serologies can become positive. When present alone or co-infecting with B. burgdorferi, persistent leukopenia is an important clue. Thrombocytopenia and elevated liver enzymes are less common, but likewise should not be ignored. Headaches, myalgias, and ongoing fatigue seem to relate to this illness, but are extremely difficult to separate from symptoms caused by Bb.

Toward the end of the 19th century, scientists began to understand the important potential for ticks to act as transmitters of disease. In the last decades of the 20th century, several tick-borne diseases have been recognized in the United States, including babesiosis, Lyme disease, and ehrlichiosis.

Ehrlichiosis is caused by several bacterial species in the genus Ehrlichia (pronounced err-lick-ee-uh) which have been recognized since 1935. Over several decades, veterinary pathogens that caused disease in dogs, cattle, sheep, goats, and horses were identified. Currently, three species of Ehrlichia in the United States and one in Japan are known to cause disease in humans; others could be recognized in the future as methods of detection improve.

In 1953, the first ehrlichial pathogen of humans was identified in Japan. Sennetsu fever, caused by Ehrlichia sennetsu, is characterized by fever and swollen lymph nodes. The disease is very rare outside the Far East and Southeast Asia, and most cases have been reported from western Japan.

In the United States, human diseases caused by Ehrlichia species have been recognized since the mid-1980s. The ehrlichioses represent a group of clinically similar, yet epidemiologically and etiologically distinct, diseases caused by Ehrlichia chaffeensis, E. ewingii, and a bacterium extremely similar or identical to E. phagocytophila. The remainder of the information on this web page will focus on the types of ehrlichiosis that occur in the United States.

Human ehrlichiosis due to Ehrlichia chaffeensis was first described in 1987. The disease occurs primarily in the southeastern and south central regions of the country and is primarily transmitted by the lone star tick, Amblyomma americanum.

Human granulocytic ehrlichiosis (HGE) represents the second recognized ehrlichial infection of humans in the United States, and was first described in 1994. The name for the species that causes HGE has not been formally proposed, but this species is closely related or identical to the veterinary pathogens Ehrlichia equi and Ehrlichia phagocytophila. HGE is transmitted by the blacklegged tick (Ixodes scapularis) and the western blacklegged tick (Ixodes pacificus) in the United States.

Ehrlichia ewingii is the most recently recognized human pathogen. Disease caused by E. ewingii has been limited to a few patients in Missouri, Oklahoma, and Tennessee, most of whom have had underlying immunosuppression. The full extent of the geographic range of this species, its vectors, and its role in human disease is currently under investigation.

DIAGNOSTIC TESTING

Testing is problematic with Ehrlichia, similar to the situation with Babesiosis. More species are known to be present in ticks than can be tested for with clinically available serologies and PCRs. In addition, serologies and PCRs are of unknown sensitivity and specificity. Standard blood smears for direct visualization of organisms in leukocytes are of low yield. Enhanced smears using buffy coats significantly raises sensitivity and will indicate a wider variety of species. Despite this, infection can be missed, so clinical diagnosis remains the primary diagnostic tool.

Again, consider this diagnosis in a Lyme Borreliosis (LB) patient not responding well to therapy.

TREATMENT

Standard treatment consists of Doxycycline, 200 mg daily for two to four weeks. Higher doses, parenteral therapy, and longer treatment durations may be needed based on the duration and severity of illness, and whether immune defects or extreme age is present. However, there are reports of treatment failure even when higher doses and long duration treatment with doxycycline is given. In such cases, consideration may be given for adding rifampin, 600 mg daily, to the regimen.

BARTONELLA

Bartonella henselae, the agent of cat scratch disease, has been found in Ixodid ticks and as a co-infection in patients with Lyme Disease. With co-infection, symptoms of Bartonella are almost impossible to distinguish from Lyme, but may include lymphadenopathy, splenomegaly, hepatomegaly, headache, encephalopathy, somnolence, flu-like malaise, weight loss, sore throat, and a papular or angiomatous rash. In acute cases, there can be hemolysis with anemia, high fever, weakened immune response, jaundice, abnormal liver enzymes, and myalgias. Endocarditis and myocarditis have been reported. More severe infections are associated with immune deficiency and possibly occurrence of opportunistic infections. As in Lyme Disease and Babesiosis,

Bartonella may be transmitted to the fetus in the infected pregnant patient. Diagnostic tests include serology, blood and CSF PCR, and biopsy of skin lesions and lymph nodes. In the co-infected Lyme patient, eradication may be difficult. Many antibiotic agents have been reported to be effective, including cephalosporins, fluoroquinolones, erythromycins, gentamicin, rifampin and streptomycin. In practice, these patients seem to do best with a combination regimen that utilizes agents that can penetrate cells. Typical combinations include an erythromycin, plus a fluoroquinolone or rifampin. Treatment progress is most commonly assessed by PCR post treatment and serial titers.

TULAREMIA

see pictures of tularemia infection at http://www.beaglesunlimited.net/rabbithunting_tularemia.htm

Tularemia is an infectious disease caused by a hardy bacterium, *Francisella tularensis*, found in animals (especially rodents, rabbits, and hares).

People can get tularemia many different ways, such as through the bite of an infected insect or other arthropod (usually a tick or deerfly), handling infected animal carcasses, eating or drinking contaminated food or water, or breathing in *F. tularensis*.

Symptoms of tularemia could include sudden fever, chills, headaches, muscle aches, joint pain, dry cough, progressive weakness, and pneumonia. Persons with pneumonia can develop chest pain and bloody spit and can have trouble breathing or can sometimes stop breathing. Other symptoms of tularemia depend on how a person was exposed to the tularemia bacteria. These symptoms can include ulcers on the skin or mouth, swollen and painful lymph glands, swollen and painful eyes, and a sore throat. Symptoms usually appear 3 to 5 days after exposure to the bacteria, but can take as long as 14 days.

Tularemia is not known to be spread from person to person, so people who have tularemia do not need to be isolated. People who have been exposed to *F. tularensis* should be treated as soon as possible. The disease can be fatal if it is not treated with the appropriate antibiotics.

A vaccine for tularemia is under review by the Food and Drug Administration and is not currently available in the United States.

TICK PARALYSIS

Tick paralysis (tick toxicosis) – one of the eight most common tickborne diseases in the United States (1) – is an acute, ascending, flaccid motor paralysis that can be confused with Guillain-Barre syndrome, botulism, and myasthenia gravis. This report summarizes the results of the investigation of a case of tick paralysis in Washington.

On April 10, 1995, a 2-year-old girl who resided in Asotin County, Washington, was taken to the emergency department of a regional hospital because of a 2-day history of unsteady gait, difficulty standing, and reluctance to walk. Other than a recent history of cough, she had been healthy and had not been injured. On physical examination, she was afebrile, alert, and active but could stand only briefly before requiring assistance. Cranial nerve function was intact. However, she exhibited marked extremity and mild truncal ataxia, and deep tendon reflexes were absent. She was admitted with a tentative diagnosis of either Guillain-Barre syndrome or postinfectious polyradiculopathy.

Within several hours of hospitalization, she had onset of drooling and tachypnea. A nurse incidentally detected an engorged tick on the girl's hairline by an ear and removed the tick. Within 7 hours after tick removal, tachypnea subsided and reflexes were present but diminished. The patient recovered fully and was discharged on April 11. The tick species was not identified.

Reported by: E Haas, D Anderson, R Neu, Asotin County Health Dept, Clarkston, Washington. N Berkheiser, MD, Saint Joseph Regional Medical Center, Lewiston, Idaho. J Grendon, DVM, P Shoemaker, J Kobayashi, MD, P Stehr-Green, DrPH, State Epidemiologist, Washington State Dept of Health. Div of Field Epidemiology, Epidemiology Program Office, CDC. http://www.cdc.gov/mmwr/preview/mmwrhtml/00040975.htm

Editorial Note: Tick paralysis occurs worldwide and is caused by the introduction of a neurotoxin elaborated into humans during attachment of and feeding by the female of several tick species. In North America, tick paralysis occurs most commonly in the Rocky Mountain and northwestern regions of the United States and in western Canada. Most cases have been reported among girls aged less than 10 years during April-June, when nymphs and mature wood ticks are most prevalent (2). Although tick paralysis is a reportable disease in Washington, surveillance is passive, and only 10 cases were reported during 1987-1995.

In the United States, this disease is associated with Dermacentor andersoni (Rocky Mountain wood tick), D. variabilis (American dog tick), Amblyomma americanum (Lone Star tick), A. maculatum, Ixodes scapularis (black-legged tick), and I. pacificus (western black-legged tick) (3,4). Onset of symptoms usually occurs after a tick has fed for several days. The pathogenesis of tick paralysis has not been fully elucidated, and pathologic and clinical effects vary depending on the tick species (4). However, motor neurons probably are affected by the toxin, which diminishes release of acetylcholine (5). In addition, experimental studies indicate that the toxin may produce a substantial decrease in maximal motor-nerve conduction velocities while simultaneously increasing the stimulating current potential necessary to elicit a response (5).

If unrecognized, tick paralysis can progress to respiratory failure and may be fatal in approximately 10% of cases (6). Prompt removal of the feeding tick usually is followed by complete recovery. Ticks can be attached to the scalp or neck and concealed by hair and can be removed using forceps or tweezers to grasp the tick as closely as possible to the point of attachment (7). Removal requires the application of even pressure to avoid breaking off the body and leaving the mouth parts imbedded in the host. Gloves should be worn if a tick must be removed by hand; hands should be promptly washed with soap and hot water after removal of a tick.

The risk for tick paralysis may be greatest for children in rural areas, especially in the Northwest, during the spring and may be reduced by the use of repellants on skin and permethrin-containing acaricides on clothing. Paralysis can be prevented by careful examination of potentially exposed persons for ticks and prompt removal of ticks. Health-care providers should consider tick paralysis in persons who reside or have recently visited tick-endemic areas during the spring or early summer and who present with symmetrical paralysis.

References

Spach DH, Liles WC, Campbell GL, Quick RE, Anderson DE, Fritsche TR. Tick-borne diseases in the United States. N Engl J Med 1993;329:936–47.

CDC. Tick paralysis – Wisconsin. MMWR 1981; 30:217–8.

CDC. Tick paralysis – Georgia. MMWR 1977; 26:311.

Gothe R, Kunze K, Hoogstraal H. The mechanisms of pathogenicity in the tick paralyses. J Med Entomol 1979;16:357–69.

Kocan AA. Tick paralysis. J Am Vet Med Assoc 1988;192:1498–500.

Schmitt N, Bowmer EJ, Gregson JD. Tick paralysis in British Columbia. Can Med Assoc J 1969;100:417–21.

Needham GR. Evaluation of five popular methods for tick removal. Pediatrics 1985;75:997–1002.

ROCKY MOUNTAIN SPOTTED FEVER (Rickettsia)

- Rocky Mountain spotted fever is a serious, generalized illness that is usually spread by the bite of an infected tick.
- Anyone who is exposed to areas where ticks live or to pets with ticks is at risk for Rocky Mountain spotted fever.
- Rocky Mountain spotted fever is treatable with antibiotics. Without treatment, the disease can be fatal.
- Rocky Mountain spotted fever can be prevented by: 1) avoiding tick bites, 2) removing attached ticks promptly, and 3) getting early diagnosis and treatment.

What is Rocky Mountain spotted fever?

Rocky Mountain spotted fever is a serious, generalized infection that is usually spread to people by the bite of infected ticks. The disease gets its name from the Rocky Mountain area where it was first identified.

What is the infectious agent that causes Rocky Mountain spotted fever?

Rocky Mountain spotted fever is caused by Rickettsia rickettsii, a specialized bacteria. Ticks infected with the organism transmit the disease to humans.

Where is Rocky Mountain spotted fever found?

Rocky Mountain spotted fever is found throughout the United States, except in Maine, Alaska, and Hawaii. Despite the name, few cases are reported from the Rocky Mountain region. Most cases occur in the southeastern United States.

Rocky Mountain spotted fever is spread by the American dog tick, the lone-star tick, and the wood tick, all of which like to live in wooded areas and tall, grassy fields. The disease is most common in the spring and summer when these ticks are active, but it can occur anytime during the year when the weather is warm.

How do people get Rocky Mountain spotted fever?

People get Rocky Mountain spotted fever from the bite of an infected tick or by contamination of the skin with the contents of an attached tick when it is removed from the skin. Rocky Mountain spotted fever is not spread from person to person, except rarely by blood transfusion.

What are the signs and symptoms of Rocky Mountain spotted fever?

People with Rocky Mountain spotted fever get a sudden fever (which can last for 2 or 3 weeks), severe headache, tiredness, deep muscle pain, chills, nausea, and a characteristic rash. The rash might begin on the legs or arms, can include the soles of the feet or palms of the hands, and can spread rapidly to the trunk or the rest of the body.

How soon after exposure do symptoms appear?

Symptoms usually begin 3 to 12 days after a tick bite.

How is Rocky Mountain spotted fever diagnosed?

The disease is diagnosed by special blood tests.

Who is at risk for Rocky Mountain spotted fever?

Anyone who is exposed to tick-infested areas or to tick-infested pets is at risk for Rocky Mountain spotted fever.

What complications can result from Rocky Mountain spotted fever?

Without prompt medical care, kidney failure and shock can lead to death.

What is the treatment for Rocky Mountain spotted fever?

Rocky Mountain spotted fever must be treated with antibiotics. Many persons with the disease need to be hospitalized.

How common is Rocky Mountain spotted fever?

Rocky Mountain spotted fever affects about 800 persons in the United States each year.

Is Rocky Mountain spotted fever a new or emerging infectious disease?

No. However, because of the seriousness of the disease, continued efforts are needed to increase awareness and encourage prevention.

How can Rocky Mountain spotted fever be prevented?

No vaccine is available to protect humans against Rocky Mountain spotted fever. The best way to avoid getting the disease is to avoid areas such as the woods or fields where ticks are found. If this is not possible, you can reduce your risk by taking these precautions:

1. Control the tick population on your property. Keep pets tick-free. Mow grass often in yards and outside fences.

2. During outside activities in wooded areas and around tall grass, wear long sleeves and long pants tucked into socks.

3. Use insecticides to repel or kill ticks. Repellents containing the compound DEET can be used on exposed skin except for the face, but they do not kill ticks and are not 100% effective in discouraging ticks from biting. Products containing permethrin kill ticks, but they cannot be used on the skin – only on clothing. When using any of these chemicals, follow label directions carefully. Be especially cautious when using them on children.

4. After outdoor activities, check yourself for ticks, and have a "buddy" check you, too. Check body areas where ticks are commonly found: behind the knees, between the fingers and toes, under the arms, in and behind the ears, and on the neck, hairline, and top of the head. Check places where clothing presses on skin.

5. Remove attached ticks immediately. Removing a tick before it has been attached for more than 4 hours greatly reduces the risk of infection. Use tweezers, and grab as closely to the skin as possible. Do not handle ticks with bare hands. Do not try to remove ticks by squeezing them, coating them with petroleum jelly, or burning them with a match.

6. After removing the tick, thoroughly disinfect the bite site, and wash your hands. See or call a doctor if you think that tick parts may remain in your skin. If you get a fever, headache, rash, or nausea within 2 weeks of a possible tick bite or exposure, see a doctor right away.

This fact sheet is for information only and is not meant to be used for self-diagnosis or as a substitute for consultation with a health-care provider. If you have any questions about the disease described above, consult a health-care provider.

8. <u>Sex and Lyme Disease</u> gives an even deeper understanding of the amazing damage Lyme disease can wreak on you or your family! This article by Dr Bransfield says it all!

<u>http://www.mentalhealthandillness.com/</u>
has several articles by Dr. Bransfield that you may find interesting.

8

SEX AND LYME DISEASE

By Robert C Bransfield, M.D.

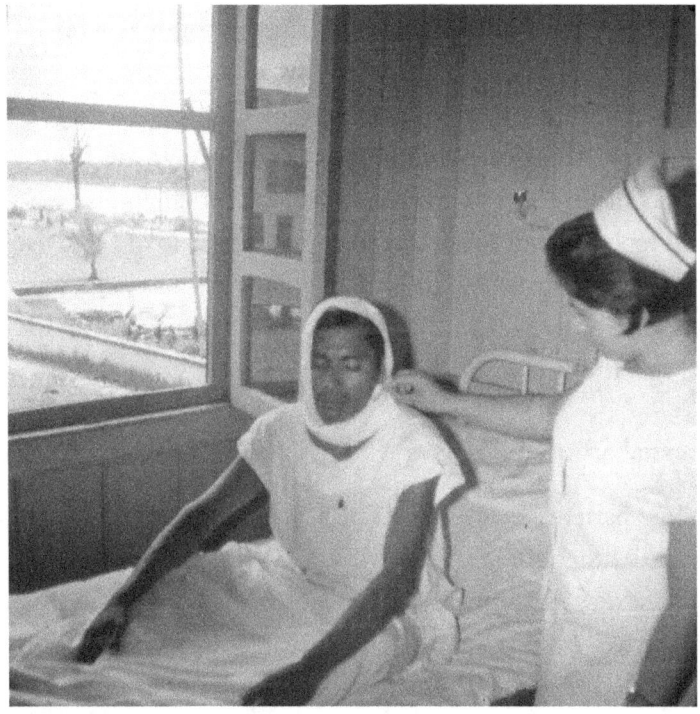

Jungle hospital with patient who is being attended by nurse. Patient is suffering from fever of unknown origin and has wrapped her head area in cloth to "protect" herself from the "bad air" that blows through the window of the room. This is a superstitious idea of native origin.

❁ ❁ ❁

How does chronic Lyme disease affect sexual functioning, and how can it be treated? Lyme can affect sexual functioning by its effect upon the central nervous system, the endocrine system, the autonomic nervous system, the peripheral nervous system, and/or the body.

It is well recognized that Borrelia burgdorferi (Bb) causes depression, obsessiveness, panic disorder, and phobias that are functions of the emotional aversive pathways of the brain. However, we can also see dysfunction of the reward pathways as well, which affect capacity for pleasure, feeding, bonding and sex. Since Lyme disease alters the aversive pathways which affect what and who we are repelled from, it is understandable that Lyme can also alter sexual attraction and behavioral patterns as well. With this in mind, I shall begin with some patient accounts and observations.

Sexual arousal:

Most patients report a decline in both libido and overall sexual functioning. Some state that their interest in sex and sexual functioning remain normal while a few report increased libido. One such patient described a greatly increased libido, but was frustrated because the multitudes of chronic Lyme disease symptom made it painful to be touched and/or hugged. Others describe increased libido associated with hypnagogic hallucinations. A patient with this symptom was described in the medical literature two years ago. She displayed sexual obsessions, sexual hallucinations, and a tendency to compulsively masturbate in a dream-like state eighteen hours per day if left undisturbed.*

Some patients develop an obsessive compulsive disorder with sexual obsessions, compulsions, intrusive images, and vivid dreams following the onset of chronic Lyme disease. Of particular interest, a few patients report a change in the content of sexual imagery. A change to more violent sexual themes is sometimes noted. This, in turn, sometimes alters sexual behavior.

Could Borrelia burgdorferi or other infectious diseases sometimes alter sexual orientation or contribute gender dysphoria, or altered patterns of sexual arousal? There is evidence that sexual functioning is altered by a number of other parasites, including Wolbachia, Spiroplasma, Rickettsia and Microsporidia. When Bb infections begin in childhood, are there some cases where it may have an effect upon sexual development? Is infectious disease one of the many factors that may affect sexual development? When changes in sexual imagery occur in adults, most are upset by the changes, which result in a decline of sexual interest. However, there are times when some individuals act out these fantasies."

*Stein Sara L., MD. Et al, American Journal of Psychiatry 153:4, April 1996, Clinical Case Conference "A 25- Year-Old Woman With Hallucinations, Hyper sexuality, Nightmares, and a Rash

"Fertility:

Patients complain of infertility with surprising frequency. Is infertility more common in chronic Lyme disease patients?

Atrophy of genitalia:

A few patients who have been infected for over ten years report atrophy of the genitalia. Males have reported atrophy of the penis and testicles, a change that is reversed by IV antibiotics. Females report lack of vaginal lubrication, painful intercourse, and anorgasmia. One female patient reported atrophy of one breast.

Anesthesia of genitalia:

On occasion, some patients complain of a loss or sensation of the genitalia. I have also seen this symptom in a few chronic fatigue patients.

Orgasm induced migraine headaches:

Although. uncommon, this is seen in chronic Lyme disease patients"

Can Lyme be sexually transmitted?

The only abstract I could find on this question is as follows:

This is an abstract presented by Dr. Bach at the International Scientific Conference on Lyme Disease, April, 2001.

RECOVERY OF LYME SPIROCHETES BY PCR IN SEMEN SAMPLES OF PREVIOUSLY DIAGNOSED LYME DISEASE PATIENTS

Dr. Gregory Bach, Do.O., P.C. 2415 North Broad Street, Colmar, PA 18915

OBJECTIVE

Lyme disease, being a spirochete with pathology similar to syphilis, is often found difficult to treat due to the spirochete invading sanctuary sites and displaying pleomorphic characteristics such as a cyst (L-form). Because a significant portion of sexually active couples present to my office with Lyme disease, with only one partner having a history of tick exposure, the question of possible secondary (sexual)vector of transmission for the spirochete warrents inquiriy.

Additionally, sexually active couples seem to have a marked propensity for antibiotic failure raising the question of sexually active couples re-infecting themselves through intimate contact.

METHODS:

Lyme spirochetes/DNA have been recovered from stored animal semen. Recovery of spirochete DNA from nursing mother's breast milk and unbilical cord blood by PCR (confirmed by culture/microscopy), have been found in samples provided to my office.

RESULTS:

Suprisingly, initial laboratory testing of semen samples provided by male Lyme patients (positive by western blot/PCR in blood) and the male sexual partner of a Lyme infected female patient were positive approximately 40% of the time. PCR recovery of Lyme DNA nucleotide sequences with microscopic confirmation of semen samples yielded positive results in 14/32 Lyme patients (13 male semen samples and 1 vaginal pap).

ALL positive semen/vaginal samples in patients with known sexual partners resulted in positive Lyme titers/PCR in their sexual partners. 3/4 positive semen patients had no or unknown sexual partners to be tested. These preliminary findings Warrant further study. Currently a statistical design study to evaluate the possibility of sexual transition of the spirochete is being undertaken.

Our laboratory studies confirm the existence of Lyme spirochetes in semen/vaginal secretions. Whether or not further clinical studies with a larger statistical group will support the hypothesis of sexual transmission remains to be seen. A retrospective clinical study is also underway.

We are reviewing the medical records, collecting semen samples of patients who were previously diagnosed with current and previously treated Lyme disease are bing asked to provide semen,pap and blood samples for extensive laboratory testing.

CONCLUSION:

With the initially impressive data, we feel the subsequent statistical sudy on the sexual transmission of the Lyme spirochete will illuminate a much broader spectrum of public health concerns associated with the disease than the originally accepted tick borne vector.

Is Lyme disease sexually transmitted? Really?

This is my personal opinion in an area of controversy. I cannot find any solid published evidence on this topic, so there is a lot of doubt in my mind as to whether or not Lyme can be readily transmitted sexually except in a very sick patient who is not on any treatment for the infection. In such a case, the sick person usually has no interest in sexual activity! Again, I happen to know entire families whose members all have the disease. How is this possible unless the family members have all been exposed to infected ticks while camping etc. and/or live in an endemic area with lots opportunity to contract this tick-borne disease.

How can it be known whether it was passed from one person to another? It would be reasonable to assume that couples could have been infected at the same time while traveling through a tick-infested area.

The case mentioned above where the Lyme DNA was found in the semen does not prove that Lyme can be transmitted via the sex organs since the urine could be where the spirochetal DNA could have originated and the urethra canal is the same one that sperm ejaculation uses. If there were live motile spirochetes in the semen, I would be more convinced of the possibility of transferring the disease sexually like syphilis or other STDs. Incidentally, syphilis is so contagious that you can be infected by kissing!

If Lyme can be transmitted sexually, I am sure there would be more cases than we already have and the epidemic would be far greater than at present.

On the other hand, we do need to make more efforts to research this possibility of sexual transfer, since we do have evidence of mother's milk being a vehicle for transferring the disease of Lyme to the offspring. I personally know of one case where the mother was bitten by an infected tick on her breast while she was still nursing her infant offspring. She developed the typical rash on the breast where the tick had bitten her and continued to nurse her baby not realizing that the tick was infected (a bulls-eye rash is almost a sure bet that the tick was carrying the Borrelia spirochete). The mother developed sever Lyme symptoms later and the child suffered from a severe case of Juvenile Arthritis which prevented him from attending full time school. So I try to keep an open mind and am willing to change my opinion as more evidence surfaces. I wish some of the "Lyme critics" out there would do the same instead of being inexcusably rigid in their set ideas!

9

NEURO-PSYCHIATRIC PROBLEMS AND LYME DISEASE:

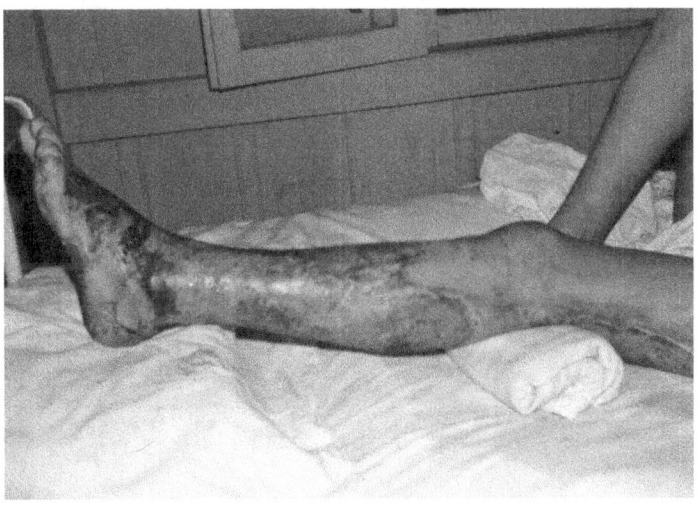

Young native with 2nd and 3rd degree burns from a gasoline explosion while repairing an electrical relay under a car.

ℜ ℜ ℜ

There is also evidence that neuro-psychiatric problems may also be caused by Lyme disease:

Canadian Lyme Disease Foundation

Rapidly progressive frontal-type dementia associated with Lyme disease. Publisher abstract: http://neuro. psychiatryonline.org/cgi/content/abstract/7/3/345
AUTHORS: Waniek C; Prohovnik I; Kaufman MA; Dwork AJ
AUTHOR AFFILIATION: New York State Psychiatric Institute, NY 10032, USA. SOURCE:
J Neuropsychiatry Clin Neurosci 1995 Summer;7(3):345-7

ABSTRACT: The authors report a case of fatal neuropsychiatric Lyme disease (LD) that was expressed clinically by progressive frontal lobe dementia and pathologically by severe subcortical degeneration. Antibiotic treatment resulted in transient improvement, but the patient relapsed after the antibiotics were discontinued. LD must be considered even in cases with purely psychiatric presentation, and prolonged antibiotic therapy may be necessary.

Psychiatric Manifestations

Brian A. Fallon, M.D.
Department of Psychiatry, College of Physicians and Surgeons of Columbia University Division of Therapeutics, New York State Psychiatric Institute, New York, New York.,

Jenifer A. Nields, M.D., Joseph J. Burrascano, M.D. Southampton Hospital, Southampton, New York., Kenneth Liegner, M.D. Northern Westchester Hospital Center, Mt. Kisco, New York. Donato DelBene, B.A. Department of Psychiatry, College of Physicians and Surgeons of Columbia University, and Division of Therapeutics, New York State Psychiatric Institute, New York, New York., Michael R. Liebowitz, M.D. Department of Psychiatry, College of Physicians and Surgeons of Columbia University, and Division of Therapeutics, New York State Psychiatric Institute, New York, New York

Reprinted from: Psychiatric Quarterly, Vol63, No 1, Spring 1992

A review of the world literature on the psychiatric manifestations of Lyme borreliosis suggests that psychiatric problems may be a prominent feature of Lyme borreliosis. The literature consists largely of case reports and small series and thus must be regarded as suggestive rather than definitive.

In 1930 a patient was described who three months after an ECM rash developed an encephalitis with psychotic symptoms and marked CSF abnormalities (34). More recently, a patient with Lyme borreliosis was described whose clinical picture was indistinguishable from an endogenous schizophrenia (35). The patient's paranoia and hallucinations remitted after one week of antibiotic treatment with ceftriazone, but afterwards the patient showed a mild organic brain syndrome.

In Europe, two recent review articles have stated that psychiatric symptoms can be a prominent feature of Lyme borreliosis, including agitated depression and psychosis (36,37). Kohler described a staging of psychiatric symptoms which parallel the neurologic ones. In stage I, fibromyalgia, painful muscular fasciculations, and mild depression may dominate the clinical picture. In stage II, a lymphocytic meningopolyneuritis may occur along with an organic psychiatric disorder, such as an organic affective syndrome or an organic personality syndrome. In stage III, chronic encephalitides and myelitides may be accompanied by severe psychiatric syndromes, such as organic psychoses, dementia, and anorexia nervosa. This staging was based on clinical observation not systematic studies.

In the United States, Pachner (38) presented two patients whose symptoms were largely psychiatric. A 12 year old boy with confirmed Lyme arthritis treated with oral antibiotics subsequently became depressed and anorexic. After being admitted to a psychiatric hospital with the diagnosis of anorexia nervosa, he was noted to have positive serologic tests for Borrelia burgdorferi. Treatment with a 14 day course of intravenous antibiotics led to a resolution of his depression and anorexia; this improvement was sustained on 3 year follow-up. A 21 year old man seropositive for Borrelia burgdorferi developed progressive confusion, agitation, disorientation, inappropriate laughter, and violent outbursts, a temporal lobe biopsy revealed spirochetes. Treatment with IV penicillin resulted in a return to normality within 3 months.

In one U.S. study of 27 patients with late neuro-borreliosis, 33% were depressed based on their scores on the Minnesota Multiphasic Personality Inventory (2). 89% of these 27 patients also had evidence of a mild encephalopathy, characterized by memory loss (81%), excessive daytime sleepiness (30%), extreme irritability (26%), and word finding difficulties (19%). Controlled studies indicate significantly more depression among patients with late Lyme borreliosis than among normal controls (20) and other chronically ill patients (39).

Confounding accurate diagnosis is the fact that many of the prominent symptoms of Lyme disease share features with depressive illness, including irritability, fatigue, emotional lability, poor concentration, memory problems, and impaired sleep (2). Ruling out Lyme disease as a cause of these depressive symptoms can be difficult because currently available serological tests are inadequate, a third of all patients do not recall a rash or tick bite, and a long quiescent period may precede the late symptoms. Even when the diagnosis of Lyme disease is clear, optimal treatment of these depressive symptoms is uncertain because in many patients the symptoms persist even after the standard 3 week course of antibiotics. Psychiatrists currently have no guidelines on how to treat these patients. While some doctors feel that depressive symptoms in the context of Lyme disease are evidence of continued disseminated infection, others believe that these represent a secondary emotional response to having a serious illness. Appropriate treatment if the former is true would consist of further antibiotics, while if the latter is true psychotherapy and/or antidepressant therapy would be the treatment of choice. Delayed additional antibiotic treatment due to an incorrect assessment of the disease process may enable an acute illness to develop into a chronic one (2).

In conclusion, further systematic study is clearly needed to better understand the prevalence and pathophysiology of psychiatric problems among patients with Lyme borreliosis and to identify optimal treatment. A critical review of the literature indicates that disturbances of mood, memory, and sleep are prominent features of this illness. Whether borrelia burgdorferi also causes psychotic disorders and eating disorders remains an open question. Neurosyphilis, also caused by a spirochete, is known to be associated with memory problems, depression, mania, psychosis, and personality changes, such as irritability, emotional lability, and apathy (40). Given the remarkable similarities between syphilis and Lyme borreliosis, it is possible that the full range of psychiatric symptoms seen in neurosyphilis may also soon be recognized as features of Lyme borreliosis.

Photophobia (sensitivity to light)

As in various other infections and/or CNS disturbances (e.g. meningitis, migraine, psittacosis, typhus, Rocky Mountain Spotted Fever), photophobia may be a prominent feature. In our sample, 70% of respondents reported photophobia. The severity of this symptom can be quite striking, and there may be variants, including idiosyncratic responses to particular kinds of light. Patients may need to wear sunglasses or glacier glasses, even indoors, even at night. Several patients reported feeling "faint" or "dizzy" in particular when exposed to fluorescent lights, making it difficult to go to supermarkets or other public places. Of note: such a patient might be referred to a psychiatrist because of what seemed like agoraphobia. Some patients have developed panic-attacks that seemed to be triggered by sound or light stimulation-especially bright lights that flicker, such as fluorescent lights-and which resolved following antibiotic treatment. others have developed nausea in response, again, to lights that flicker: fluorescent lights, TV or computer screens, strobe lights during EEG testing or the headlights of cars moving in the opposite line of traffic. The hyper-sensitivity to light can be incapacitating or merely uncomfortable. It may preclude driving at night or going outdoors during the day or it may make what are normally routine or even pleasurable activities seem noxious.

Sound Sensitivity

A more distinctive, somewhat less common but often very intense symptom, reported in 48% of our sample, is hypersensitivity to and/or idiosyncratic responses to sound stimulation. One boy developed sound sensitivity so severe that ordinary conversation was deafening to him; he wore head phones and put pillows over his head to block out the sound. To one woman even the sound of another person's breathing seemed unbearably loud. In her case, the sound sensitivity also included vertigo, nausea and nystagmus in response to sounds. Any sudden sound, like the phone ringing, and certain household sounds, like the running of tap water, could cause her to fall or retch. This peculiar short-circuiting of the inner ear's auditory and vestibular functions is known as the Tullio phenomenon. This phenomenon has been deemed pathognomonic for syphilis (43) but, as it appears, can occur in Lyme disease as well (41), and thus provides one more example of the "new great imitator," Lyme disease, imitating the old "great imitator," syphilis (1).

Sensory Hyperacusis (increased hearing which could be irritating)

As previously reported in illnesses caused by other species of borrelia (44), hypersensitivity can occur in other sensory modalities as well: touch, taste and smell. Abnormalities of taste and smell occurred in 33% and 25% of our sample, respectively. Foods may taste abnormally sour or bitter, smells may seem overly intense and noxious. Alterations in the perception or processing of other kinds of sensory stimulation occur also. One patient, before she realized she was ill with Lyme disease, noticed one day that her car was vibrating with unusual violence. She took the car emergently in to a mechanic, thinking that the shock absorbers were shot or the ball bearings loose and that it would be dangerous to continue to drive the car in that condition. As it turned out, there was nothing wrong with the car. The problem was in the patient who had suddenly and unwittingly developed a heightened sensitivity to vibrations. She subsequently became alert to this heightened vibration sense in other contexts as well. When the diagnosis of Lyme disease was finally made, this symptom, along with other, more common symptoms of Lyme disease, resolved with antibiotic treatment.

Extreme Irritability and/or Emotional Lability

Many patients reported mood and behavioral changes during the course of their illness. In our sample, 64% of patients reported increased irritability and/or emotional lability in association with symptoms suggestive of meningeal irritation: neck stiffness and headache. The mood and behavior changes are often so severe and pervasive as to constitute a personality change. Sudden, intense irritability is most often triggered by sensory stimulation in patients who are acutely sensitive to sound, touch or light but may also occur unprovoked and seemingly inexplicably. One man, acutely sensitive to sound, was so intensely bothered by the noise his three-year-old son was making that he picked him up and shook him in a sudden and unprecedented fit of violence. His wife was shocked and alarmed by this behavior, as was the patient himself. A woman, typically reserved and eager to please, became uncontrollably irritable one day at work and found herself yelling at her boss in a most uncharacteristic fashion. Others have found themselves bursting into tears, sometimes several times a day, on what seems like very little provocation.

Word Reversals When Speaking and/or Letter Reversals When Writing

These odd, idiosyncratic but quite common symptoms were reported in 69% of our sample. Patients with no prior history of dyslexia have found themselves writing letters backwards, reversing numbers or routinely reversing the first and second letters of a word. One patient recalls also switching her shoes: putting the left shoe on the right foot and the right shoe on the left foot before she realized her mistake. This patient also experienced what might be understood as reversals in temporal sequencing: for instance, saying the word "tomorrow" when she meant "yesterday" and vice versa.

Spatial Disorientation

Reported in 57% of our sample. A not uncommon scenario is of a patient who, recalling no rash or flu-like symptoms, had experienced some aches and pains and/or memory problems but had not paid much attention to these symptoms until he found himself, on two consecutive days, lost in his own neighborhood, on his way home from work. Such a scenario suggests a disorder of topographic orientation and geographic memory such as may be seen among patients with parietal lobe dysfunction (45). Patients have reported other behaviors as well which seem to relate to disturbances of the body-environmental schemata. A young woman described repeatedly bumping into things on the left side of her body, dropping things from her left hand despite having no weakness in that hand and occasionally placing objects, such as a milk carton, several inches short of a table edge with the result that they would fall to the floor. These difficulties remitted completely following adequate antibiotic treatment.

Fluctuations in Symptoms

This can be one of the most frustrating and perplexing aspects of the illness. A patient with late-stage Lyme disease might feel totally drained one day, the next day be able to function almost normally and the day after experience such mental confusion as to be unable to focus on even the simplest of tasks. Sometimes the fluctuations may be brought on by exertion or stress or exposure to sensory stimuli or by the initiation of antibiotic treatment, but sometimes no explanation can be found. The fluctuations make it impossible for patients to make plans, and may make it seem to friends, teachers, family members or even the patients themselves as if the symptoms were somehow under voluntary control or as if they were hysterical in origin. Of course psychological factors, too, can influence symptomatology, but fluctuations are typical regardless of mental state.

Such vicissitudes raise a particular problem in children who may experience fluctuating cognitive impairments: short-term memory problems, word-finding difficulties, dyslexia, problems with calculations or inability to concentrate. School systems are by and large unaware of the cognitive aspects of late-stage Lyme disease and, in particular, of the ways in which cognitive impairments may fluctuate from day to day in a given child. Teachers may assume the child is just moody or uncooperative. Family dynamics, too, may be complicated by confused expectations of the sick member, and resentments may build when a person's functional status, mood and ability to participate in family life seem inexplicably erratic. Patients and family members alike find it difficult to have their hopes raised repeatedly by a transient clinical improvement, only to be slapped down again by a recrudescence of debilitating symptoms. Even with treatment, recovery from late-stage Lyme disease is most often a lengthy process involving significant fluctuations in symptoms even in the context of overall improvement.

Worsening of Symptoms During Antibiotic Treatment

Nearly half of the patients in our sample reported a transient worsening of neuropsychiatric symptoms during the first few days of antibiotic treatment. The worsening of symptoms during initiation of antibiotic treatment is thought to be a variant of the Herxheimer reaction as seen in the treatment of syphilis (33). In Lyme disease, however, this Herxheimer-like reaction can be quite prolonged-lasting a few days or longer-and can be frightening to patients who are expecting a resolution, not a worsening, of their symptoms. The reaction can sometimes be difficult to distinguish from an allergic reaction to the medicine, a distinction with obvious and crucial treatment implications.

This Herxheimer-like reaction may be experienced as a worsening of psychiatric symptoms: some patients in our sample experienced panic attacks for the first and only time when starting on antibiotics. Others have reported an intensification of depressive symptoms, suicidality or anxiety. Many reported an increased startle response and photophobia during the first few days of antibiotic treatment.

Uncertainty as to Diagnosis and Treatment

A great deal is unknown about Lyme disease at this point in time, and experts disagree regarding its diagnosis and management. Some patients remain seronegative, for a variety of reasons (some known, some unknown) (30) and therefore remain undiagnosed and untreated for long periods of time. The medical literature now documents that some patients, even following what has been presumed to be adequate treatment, go on to develop late-stage symptoms, sometimes months or years later (2). Even now, some doctors think that so-called seronegative Lyme disease is fairly common and others that it is virtually nonexistent. Some doctors believe that prolonged antibiotic treatment may be necessary in late Lyme disease (33,46), and others, emphasizing the less specific symptoms of late Lyme disease (similar to fibromyalgia or chronic fatigue syndrome), consider such treatment in many cases to be excessive and unreasonable (47). Patients may be told that Lyme disease is easily curable with antibiotics and that further concern about it is a matter of "Lyme anxiety" (48); from other sources, they may learn that Lyme infection in some cases may lead to a chronic, severely debilitating, perhaps irreversible disease (2). Such manifold uncertainties as to diagnosis, treatment and prognosis at this stage in the history of Lyme disease put the patient in a difficult position. The patient may get conflicting advice from reputable sources and not know what to do. He may be told that his symptoms are not related to Lyme disease. He may be told there is no medical cause for his complaints and be referred to a psychiatrist. And, especially since Lyme disease may in fact involve the brain and manifest as depression or confusion or irritability, it may be hard not only for the clinician, but also for the patient himself to recognize the effects of the disease as against his emotional reactions to it. Some patients, who have subsequently been effectively treated, have said that, prior to being diagnosed, they had feared they were just going crazy.

CONCLUSION

In most cases, Lyme disease, when treated early, is a mild illness with no long-term sequelae. When first identified in its later stages, however, some of the symptoms of the illness may be less responsive to antibiotic treatment, resulting in a disabling, chronic disorder. From the foregoing clinical vignettes, it should be clear that Lyme disease, particularly when it involves the central nervous system, can in some patients be an extremely debilitating, bizarre, terrifying and perplexing disease. It can present in a great variety of ways, and the symptoms can fluctuate dramatically and unpredictably. At the same time, there are patterns to its emergence that can suggest the diagnosis in cases where laboratory indices are inconclusive. Much uncertainty surrounds the diagnosis and treatment of Lyme disease at this stage in its history, and such uncertainty adds to the distress that the illness causes for patients. Lyme disease is aptly called the "new great imitator," and it can imitate psychiatric disorders no less than medical ones. Psychiatrists working in endemic areas are well-advised, then, to keep Lyme disease in mind as part of their differential diagnosis for a broad range of disorders including, for instance, panic attacks, somatization disorder, depression, and dementia, especially in cases that are atypical or otherwise suggestive of systemic disease. It should be borne in mind also that new clinical manifestations of Lyme disease are still being discovered and described. In cases of known Lyme disease, it is important for psychiatrists to take a comprehensive approach to treatment as so many aspects of the patient's life-physical, emotional, cognitive, familial, sexual, social and occupational-may be significantly affected by the illness. --

ACKNOWLEDGMENT

Supported in part by NIMH Research Fellowship to Dr. Fallon.Address correspondence to Brian A. Fallon, M.D., New York State Psychiatric Institute, 722 West 168th Street, Box 13, New York, New York 10032., ----------------
----

REFERENCES

1. Pachner AR. Borrelia burgdorferi in the Nervous System: the New "Great Imitator." In Lyme Disease and Related Disorders. Annals New York Academy of Sciences 539: 56–64, 1988. 2. Logigian EL, Kaplan RF, Steere AC. Chronic neurologic manifestations of Lyme disease. NEJM 323: 1438-1444, 1990. 3.White DJ, Chang HG, Benach JL, et al. The geographic spread and temporal increase of the Lyme disease epidemic. JAMA 266: 1230–1236.1991. 4. Burgdorfer W. Lyme borreliosis: ten years after discovery of the etiologic agent, Borrelia burgdorferi. Infection 19: 257–262.1991. 5. Magnarelli LA. Laboratory Diagnosis of Lyme disease. Rheumatic Disease Clinics of North America. 15: 735–745, 1989. 6. Schmid GP. The global distribution of Lyme disease. Rev Infect Dis 7:41–50, 1986. 7. Weber K, et al. Erythema Migrans Disease and related disorders. Yale J Biol Med 57: 13–21, 1984. 8. Afzelius A. Erythema Chronicum Migrans. Acta Derm Venereol 2: 120–125, 192l. 9. Garin, Bujadoux: Paralysie par les tiques. J Med Lyon 71: 765–767.1922. 10. Bannwarth A: Chronische lymphocytare meningitis,

entzundliche polyneuritis and "rheumtisumes." Arch Psychiatr Nervenkr 113: 284-376, 1941. 11. Scrimenti RJ. Erythema chronicum migrans. Arch Dermatol 102: 104-105, 1970. 12. Steere AC, Malawista SE, Hardin JA. et al: Erythema chronicum migrans and Lyme arthritis. Ann Int Med 86: 685-698.1977. 13. Asbrink B. Hovmark A, Hederstedt B. The spirochetal etiology of acrodermatitis chronica atrophicans Herxheimer. Acta Derm Venereol 64: 506-512, 1984. 14. Pachner AR, Steere AC. The triad of neurologic manifestations of Lyme disease: meningitis, cranial neuritis. and radiculoneuritis. Neurology 35: 47-53. 1985. 15. Finkel MF. Lyme disease and its neurologic complications. Arch Neurol 45: 99-104, 1988 16. Halperin JJ. Nervous System Manifestations of Lyme Disease. Rheumatic Disease Clinics of North America. 15: 635-647, 1989. 17. Reznick JW, Braunstein DB, Walsh RI, Smith Cr, Wolfson PM, Gierke IW, Gorelkin I, Chandler RW. Lyme carditis. Electrophysiologic and histopathologic study. Am J Med 5: 923-927, 1986. 18. Stanek G, Klein J, Bittner R, Glogar D. Isolation of Borrelia burgdorferi from the myocardium of a patient with long-standing cardiomyopathy. NEJM 322: 249-252, 1990. 19. Halperin JJ, Pass HL, Anand AK, Luft BJ. Volkman DJ, Dattwyler RJ. Nervous system abnormalities in Lyme disease. Annals NY Acad Sciences 539: 24-34, 1988. 20. Krupp LB, Masur D, Schwartz J, Coyle PK. Langenbach LJ. Fernquist SK, Jandorf L, Halperin JJ. Cognitive functioning in late Lyme borreliosis. Arch Neurol 48: 1125-1129, 1991. 21. Steere AC, Duray PH, Danny JH, et al: Unilateral blindness caused by infection with Lyme disease spirochete, Borrelia burgdorferi. Ann Int Med 103: 382-384, 1985. 22. Halperin JJ, Kaplan GP, Brazinsky S et al: Immunologic reactivity against Borrelia burgdorferi in patients with motor neuron disease. Arch Neurol 47: 686-594.1990. 23. Clavelou P, Beytout J, Vernay D, et al: Neurologic manifestations of Lyme disease in the northern part of the Auvergne. Neurol 39 (suppl 1): 350, 1989. 24. MacDonald AB, Miranda JM. Concurrent neocortical borreliosis and Alzheimer's disease. Human Pathology 18: 750-761, 1987. 25. Reik L, Smith L, Khan A. et al. Demyelinating encephalopathy in Lyme disease. Neurology 35: 267-269, 1985. 26. Kohler J, Kern U,. Kaper J, Rhese-Kupper B, Thoden U. Chronic central nervous system involvement in Lyme borreliosis. Neurology 863-867, 1988. 27. Kohlhepp W, Kuhn W, Kruger H. Extrapyramidal features in central Lyme borreliosis. Eur Neurol 29: 150-155, 1989. 28. Ackerman R, Rhese-Kupper B, Gollmer E, Schmidt R. Chronic neurologic manifestations of Erythema migrans borreliosis. In Lyme Disease and Related Disorders. Annals NY Acad Science. 539: 16-23, 1988. 29. Lavoie PE, Lattner BP, Duray PH, Malawista SE, Barbour AG, Johnson RC. Culture positive, seronegative, traneplacental Lyme borreliosis infant mortality. IV Int. Conf. Lyme borreliosis 1990 (abstract). 30. Dattwyler RJ, Volman DJ, Luft BJ, et al. Seronegative Lyme disease. NEJM 319:1441-1446, 1988. 31. Keller TL, Halperin JJ, Whitman M, PCR detection of Borrelia burgdorferi DNA in cerebrospinal fluid of Lyme neuroborreliosis patients. Neurology 42: 32-42, 1992. 32.

Rahn DW, Malawista SE, Lyme disease: recommendations for diagnosis and treatment. Ann Intern Med 114: 472-481, 1991. 33. Burrascano J. Late-stage Lyme: treatment options and guidelines. Int Med 10:102-10, 1989. 34. Hellerstron M. Erythema chronicum migrans Afzelii. Acta Derm Venereol (Stockh) 11:305-321, 1930. (referenced in Kohler et al: Neurology 38: 863-867, 1988) 35. Barnett W, Sigmund D. Roelcke U, Mundt C. Endogenous paranoid-hallucinatory syndrome caused by Borrelia encephalitis. Nervenarzt 62: 446-7, 1991. 36. Omasits M, Seiser A, Brainin M.Recurrent and relapsing borreliosis of the nervous system. Wiener klinische wochenschrift 102: 4-12, 1990. 37. Kohler VJ. Lyme disease in neurology and psychiatry. Fortchr 108:191-194, 1991. 38. Pachner AR. Central Nervous System Manifestations of Lyme Disease. Arch Neurol 46:790-795, 1989. 39. Fallon BA, Nields JA, DelBene D, Saoud J. Wilson K, Liebowitz MR. Depression and Lyme dissease: a controlled survey. American Psychiatric Association. 145 Meeting, 1992. (Abstract). 40. Rundell JR, Wise MG. Neurosyphilis: a psychiatric perspective. Psychospomatics 26: 287-295, 1985. 41. Nields JA, Kveton JF. Tullio phenomenon and seronegative Lyme borreliosis. Lancet 338:128-129, 1991. 42. Preac-Mrusic V, Weber K, Pfister W, et al. Survival of Borrelia burgdorferi in antibiotically treated persons with Lyme borreliosis. Infection 17:355, 1989. 43. Schuknecht HF. Pathology of the Ear. Harvard University Press, Cambridge: p 133. 1974. 44. Felsenfeld O. Borrelia. Warren Green Press, St. Louis: p. 105, 1971. Adams RD, Victor M. Principles of

Neurology. 4th Edition. McGraw Hill, NY: p362-366, 1989. 45. Lavoie PE. Lyme Disease (Lyme Borreliosis). In Conn's Current Therapy 1991. 46. Rakel RE, ed. WB Saunders: 1991. 47. Sigal LH. Summary of the first 100 patients seen at a Lyme disease referral center. Amer J Med 88: 577-581, 1990. 48. Lettau L. Lime vs Lyme Disease. Ann Int Med 115: 157, 1991.

{My comments : *Hope you enjoyed looking up all the above references! I am still working on doing the same!*}

The following extract is for 'further details' on variety of symptoms:

"Many patients are told that they have Multiple Sclerosis (MS) because of brain MRI findings or a spinal tap was positive for oligoclonal bands (OCB) or myelin basic protein (MBP). The medical literature is quite emphatic that MRI does not reliably distinguish between MS an LD because there is too much overlap in their supposedly distinct appearance and location of plaques. Plaques have been detected with both disorders in the brain and spinal cord. OCB's and MBP are non-specific markers for demyelination (loss of sheath around nerves) and do not signify a cause of the demyelination. In Miklossy's study above, senile plaques stained avidly for Bb spirochetes. Vincent Marshall reviewed the MD literature in Medical Hypothesis (Vol 25: 89-92, 1988) and advances the notion that LD is causing MS! His survey revealed that multiple studies prior to 1951 were able to demonstrate spirochetes in the spinal fluid of MS patients (by inoculation into animals and on silver stain of CNS tissues). Dr. Coyle has documented the presence of antibodies to Bb in MS patients (Neurology Vol. 39:760-763, 1989). The encephalopathy attributed to MS is very reminiscent of LD. Both MS and LD are associated with sinusitis (Lancet, 1986). Dr. Leigner has reported a case of LD which fulfilled all criteria for MS. The epidemiology of MS and the geographic distribution parallels that of LD. The symptoms of both LD and MS can be aggravated if the patient takes a hot bath. Anecdotally, patients with LD, <u>who previously had been identified as MS, responded to antibiotic therapy</u>."

"Eye related problems in LD are commonplace and can include conjunctivitis, ocular myalgias, keratitis, episcleritis, optic neuritis, pars planitis, uveitis, iritis, transient or permanent blindness, temporal arteritis, vitritis and periorbital edema (Jacqueline MS; Ibid). Horner's syndrome, ocular myasthenia gravis, and an Argyll-Robertson pupil are also reported. Optic neuritis has been observed to become recurrent or intractable after treatment with steroids. Given the earlier remarks about the detrimental effects of steroids on LD, recidivous optic neuritis may be due to occult LD"

10

DO PEOPLE DIE FROM LYME DISEASE?

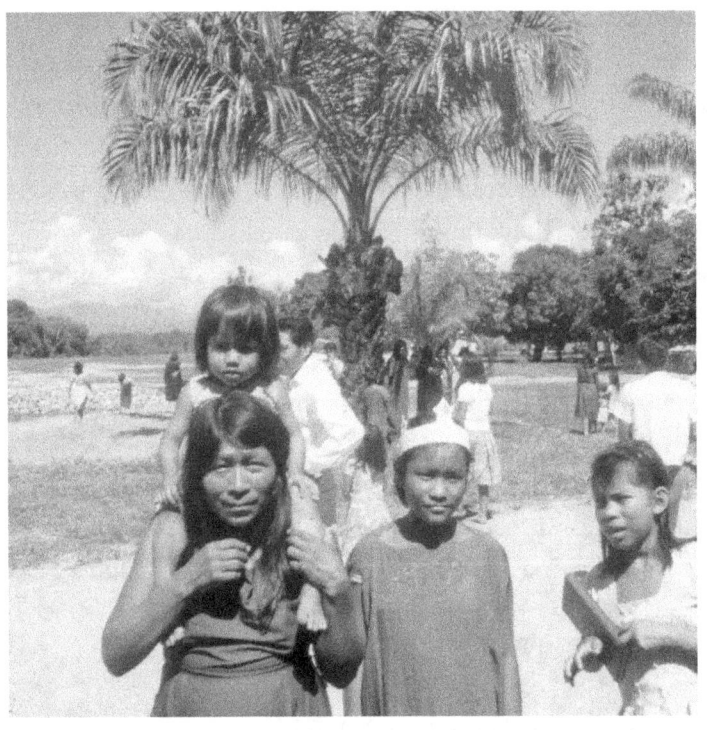

Natives living in the Amazon jungle of Peru

❃ ❃ ❃

Some people rightfully ask the above question since the cure seems so remote to most victims. Yes! People do die from Lyme disease but the disease on the death certificate is usually another name like: Multiple Sclerosis, Alzheimers, Amyotrophic Lateral Sclerosis, or perhaps Suicide secondary to the victim's inability to cope with the long term pain, or disabling symptoms that can make life "not worth living". Accidents do occur due to the victims' inability to avoid obstacles and difficulties in maintaining their balance. Vehicular accidents caused by sudden blurring of vision due to extreme light sensitivy, and a plethora of symptoms leading to related syndromes causing death.

Here is a report I received from a News outlet some months ago: The father of the deceased was a well known Seventh-day Adventist who wrote stories for children and was a renowned children's.story-teller in the SDA denomination. Many of his character-building stories have been published by the denomination.

Tue Jun 6, 2006 9:55 am (PST)
This article was sent to you via eLibrary from ProQuest Information and Learning. http://elibrary. bigchalk. com

METROPOLITAN; OBITUARIES;

The Washington Times 06-03-2006
Peter Edgar Hare, 73, Carnegie scientist

Peter Edgar Hare, noted scientist at the District"s Carnegie Institution, died May 5 at the Port Orange Christian Adult Care Home in Port Orange, Fla., following a long battle with Lyme disease. He was 73.

Mr. Hare was born April 14, 1933, in Maymyo, Burma, where his parents served as missionaries for the Seventh-day Adventist Church.

He received his bachelor's degree in chemistry from Pacific Union College in Angwin, Calif., in 1954 and earned a master's degree from the University of California at Berkeley, in 1955.

For the next three years, Mr. Hare worked as a chemistry instructor at Pacific Union.

He then studied at the California Institute of Technology and graduated with a doctorate in organic geochemistry in 1962. His dissertation, on the amino acids and proteins from carbonate minerals found in the shells of modern and fossil mussels, was published in Science magazine in 1963.

Mr. Hare's work attracted the attention of Phillip H. Abelson, who was then the director of the Carnegie Institution of Washington's Geophysical Laboratory. The two scientists corresponded for several years until Mr. Hare was invited to join the laboratory's scientific staff in 1963.

During his early years at the laboratory, Mr. Hare set up a new instrument to measure amino acids. His first paper on the development of new methodology for amino acid analysis appeared in 1966 in a publication of the Federation of the American Society for Experimental Biology.

In 1968, Mr. Hare and Mr. Abelson published the first paper on the discovery of left and right-handed amino acids in fossil shells. Mr. Hare used this information to develop a process for accurately dating ancient shells and bones.

For the rest of his career, Mr. Hare focused on studying the conversion of amino acids from left to right-handed and using the amino acid age-dating technique to date early man in North America, early human evolution in Africa and the geological progression of Arctic climates.

Mr. Hare, whose laboratory became the training ground for many young scientists, also was involved in searching for signs of life on the first rocks that came from the moon. He found some evidence for amino acids in lunar samples and published his findings in Science in 1971.

In 1979, Mr. Hare co-authored a landmark paper on new techniques for measuring left and right-handed amino acids. He and fellow author Emanuel-Av from the Weizmann Institute of Science in Israel then obtained a patent on their invention.

Mr. Hare and his wife, Patti, lived in the District"s Van Ness neighborhood when he retired from the Carnegie Institution in 1998.

In addition to his wife, Mr. Hare"s other survivors include a daughter, Carol Pack, of Laurel; a son, Calvin Hare of Orlando, Fla.; a brother, Leonard Hare of Berrien Springs, Mich., and three grandchildren.

Memorial donations can be made to the P.E. Hare Scholarship Fund at the Pacific Union College Advancement Office,

1 Angwin Ave., Angwin, Calif. 94508.

Copyright © 2006 News World Communications, Inc.

The following is a brief local Angwin newspaper announcing the same obituary from a local standpoint....

THE ANGWIN REPORTER

Duane L. Cronk, Publisher   May 18, 2006

Geologist Hare Dies

One of the most illustrious PUC graduates, Peter Hare, died last week in a nursing home in Florida. Peter, the son of Eric B. Hare, a renowned story teller, was an expert in the science of dating. He worked for the Carnegie Institute in Washington, D.C., for many years. He made national news as the scientist who was given the task of dating the moon rocks brought back to earth by Neil Armstrong in 1969. His wife, Patti, also grew up in Angwin

Since I do have a number of Seventh-day Adventist friends who would have known about this gentleman, I thought this announcement would be helpful since many

SDAs – my friends included – might not have heard of Peter Hare's passing. They may also be interested in donating to the P.E. Hare Scholarship Fund at the Pacific Union College Advancement Office,

There are many deaths today that are directly due to the complications of Lyme disease and its co-infections. The various diagnoses that are written on the death certificate is rarely Lyme disease. That is why the above obituary was shown which distinctly gives the reason for death.

Most Lyme patients who finally expire usually have diagnosis as heart failure, fatal cardiac arrythmias, Alzheimer's, ALS, Parkinson's, or in my Dad's case, "unknown."

If the truth were known, there would be many more obituaries that stated the real cause of death and not just the complications of the disease.

This subject brings to mind a retired dentist and friend who was my host on December 25th,2007 which just happens to be my birthday month. It was that evening of the 25th while I was visiting my wife's family members in Southern California that I was so completely taken by surprise as my host came into to the living room supporting himself with a walker as he shuffled slowly to be seated at the dinner table. Both he and his wife invited my wife and me over for supper that evening and we were so very happy to see them after many years of not having made contact. He looked me right in the eye without blinking once, and then he started talking in a low-pitched voice that sounded like sand in a slow motion wind tunnel. "Gordon, I have

Parkinson's and my neurologist is quite a famous specialist". I looked into my friend's eyes and marveled how difficult it was for him to speak with that hoarse, sandy voice. After listening to a series of my questions he then related his experience of years ago. About 10 years ago he was bitten by a tick which caused a "bulls-eye" rash on his body. He saw a physician since he felt the rash was an infection. The physician treated him with antibiotics for approximately 10 days after which the rash finally disappeared. Everything seemed ok after that episode. Finally, as the years slipped by, my friend began having other symptoms which finally were assigned to the diagnosis of Parkinson's syndrome! I don't believe that anyone of his physicians have ever gone that far back in my friend's history. I finally recommended testing (via his personal physician) for possible tick borne disease. If my friend finally dies, what will be his diagnosis?

This reminded me of the 65 year-old gentleman in Texas who was bedridden and wheelchair-bound due to his "Parkinson's" diagnosis for the past 15 years. He also had Bell's Palsy! His doctor had done all the testing possible without even considering tick-borne diseases. After all, which physician would think of that even today when the patient has all the signs and symptoms of Parkinson's syndrome!

To make a long story short, my friend in Texas spent 6 weeks in two 3 week sessions at a "Health Clinic" where he was treated with hot whirpool baths – hot enough to raise his body temperature to 103 degrees F for 30 minutes each day for 4 days/week. At the end of the 3rd week, my 65 year-old Texan was riding a bicycle and walking 1-3 miles daily. One month later he is still doing quite well and has not started any antibiotic therapy as yet! More about this later.

11

ANIMALS AND LYME DISEASE

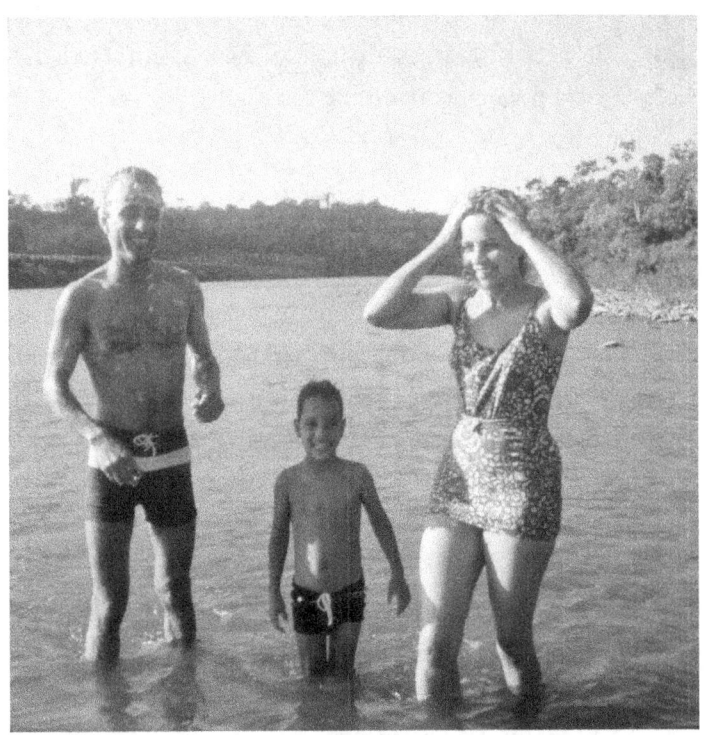

The author and his family bathing in the Unini River which flows into the Amazon River. This is a very remote area in the Peruvian jungle where we participated in medical care of the local people for a few weeks.

❦ ❦ ❦

Canadian Lyme Disease Foundation Lyme disease a concern for dogs

Published: Sunday, May 22nd, 2005

If caught in early stages, the disease is easily cured.

YOUNGSTOWN — Lyme disease is a dangerous threat to dogs, but few Ohio dog owners are aware of the risks their pets run, signs their dogs have contracted the bacteria, and means to avoid the disease.

Humans are also susceptible to Lyme disease.

A 2005 survey of 1,000 U.S. dog owners and 100 Ohio dog owners conducted by IDEXX Laboratories, Inc., with support from the American Lyme Disease Foundation, found only 3 percent of Ohio owners were concerned about their dogs contracting the disease.

The Spring Canine Lyme Disease Advisory said dogs may develop heart disease, central nervous system disorders or fatal kidney disease after being infected with the bacteria.

The ALDF said Lyme disease is easily cured if diagnosed and treated with antibiotics in its early stages; rarely does Lyme disease result in permanent damage.

Local cases

Dr. Donald K. Allen, of Dr. Donald K. Allen Veterinarian Inc. in Youngstown, said Lyme disease is present in Ohio.

"I've had maybe half a dozen cases test positive in this area in the past two years. One dog probably contracted the disease near Presque Isle, so I'd say the entire Northeast corner has it," he said.

Lyme disease is carried by deer ticks. Dr. Allen said Northeast Ohio has a fairly high deer population, which contributes to the prevalence of Lyme disease.

Dogs contract Lyme disease only from deer tick bites. The disease is caused by Borrelia burgdorferi, a bacterium that lives in the gut of deer ticks. Deer tick season is from September through April, Allen said, although dogs can contract the disease any time.

According to the Centers for Disease Control, Lyme disease has a typical incubation period of seven to 14 days, but it may be as short as three days or as long as 30 days.

Symptoms

The Spring Canine Lyme Disease Advisory listed symptoms including recurrent arthritis, lameness that lasts three to four days, loss of appetite, depression, reluctance to move, elevated temperature, fatigue and swollen lymph nodes. However, Dr. Allen said some dogs show no symptoms when they contract the disease.

Dr. Allen said ticks migrate to the head and neck area. He recommended Ticktrol, a collar with active ingredient amitraz, and topical treatments Frontline Top Spot and Advantix to help control ticks. There is also a Lyme disease vaccine.

Dr. Allen said dogs are tested for Lyme disease when they are tested for heartworm and Ehrlichia.

Humans also are susceptible to Lyme disease from deer tick bites. The CDC listed symptoms including elevated temperature, fatigue, muscle aches and characteristic "bull's-eye" rash.

Prevention

To help prevent contracting Lyme disease, Dr. Allen recommended wearing long pants and long-sleeve shirts, and tucking pant bottoms into socks. He said light-colored clothing helps make dark ticks more visible, and suggested hiking partners check each other for ticks.

Dr. Allen suggested visiting the vet or doctor if it is possible Lyme disease is contracted. However, he cautioned that tests can sometimes be falsely negative because of the incubation period.

Make dark ticks more visible, and suggested hiking partners check each other for ticks.

Lyme disease and man's canine companions

Pets and humans share the risks and the symptoms
Thursday, June 16, 2005
By JOHN A. ZUKOWSKI
The Express-Times

Veterinarian Geoffrey Wright examines many kinds of dogs.

But there's something that one out of every four dogs Wright sees in his Bethlehem office has in common.

"They've been exposed to Lyme disease," he says.

Just 4 percent of dogs he sees develop full-blown cases of Lyme disease. But the rate of dogs being exposed to Lyme disease has skyrocketed in recent years, he says.

"There are areas south of us where it's 75 percent and other areas in Connecticut where it's 100 percent where every dog has had some exposure," he says.

In New Jersey, where Lyme disease is a growing problem in Warren and Hunterdon Counties, the exposure rate for dogs isn't that high. But it's generally higher than in Pennsylvania.

"We're seeing about a 40 percent exposure rate," says veterinarian Vincent Zaccheo of Warren Animal Hospital in Lopatcong Township.

Because of the combination of a high deer population and an abundance of areas where ticks thrive, Pennsylvania and New Jersey are two high-risk states for Lyme disease, according to the U.S. Centers for Disease Control and Prevention.

As is the case with humans, a dog contracts the disease by being bitten by a deer tick.

But while more people are checking themselves for ticks after being outdoors, some dog owners don't realize dogs can contract the disease, too. So they may not check for ticks on their dogs.

Some dog owners also may think Lyme disease just affects dogs on farms or in the country. But that's not the case.

"It's certainly not just isolated to country dogs," Zaccheo says. "We've even seen it in dogs from New York City who have picked it up in Central Park on a walk."

In some cases, humans contract Lyme disease from a tick a dog carried into their home.

"People can't contract Lyme disease directly from a dog that has it," Zaccheo says. "But a tick can drop off a dog onto a bed or a couch and someone can contract if from a pet that way."

Some symptoms of Lyme disease in dogs are the same as in humans. However, symptoms in dogs can be more difficult to detect.

Once infected, a rash often forms. However, the rash usually isn't seen because it because it's under the dog's fur. So dog owners must look for other symptoms.

"The most common symptoms are limping, joint pain and arthritic-type symptoms," Zaccheo says. "But we all see dogs coming in that have symptoms of a high fever and that are lethargic and just not feeling well."

In a few cases, Lyme disease can be fatal to dogs. That happens when the disease affects the kidneys. That's more common in younger dogs than older dogs.

However, local veterinarians emphasize dog owners can reduce the odds of dogs contracting Lyme disease.

A number of preventative products are available, including vaccinations, collars and ointments. Veterinarians often also advise dog owners to be cautious where they walk their dogs. They also instruct homeowners to mow the lawn and clear debris to reduce the chance of ticks thriving around the home.

Dogs aren't the only animals that contract Lyme disease. Horses, birds and cattle also have become infected with it. Cats that go outside occasionally pick up the disease.

"But cats are most fastidious in their cleaning and grooming so Lyme disease isn't such a problem for cats," Zaccheo says.

Local veterinarians say Lyme disease in cats still lags far behind the cases of dogs contracting it. But along with more dogs being exposed to Lyme disease, dog owners are also becoming aware of it. So they're doing something to help reduce the risk.

"These days it takes a two-pronged approach of preventive measures with the dogs and doing things outside the home to help keep ticks away," Wright says.

Horses:

The symptoms of Lyme disease in horses are: chronic weight loss, sporadic lameness, laminitis (inflammation of the tissues inside the hoof wall), low grade fever, weight loss, swollen joints, muscle tenderness, eye inflammation, and stiffness. Neurological signs are depression, dysphagia (difficulty swallowing), head tilt and encephalitis, and can be observed in chronic or late stage cases. Behavioral changes are more difficult to determine, but can present as a "changed attitude", unwillingness to work (perhaps due to pain), and irritability. Foal mortality is a possibility.

Equine disease is diagnosed by determining if the animal is living in an endemic area, history of actual tick exposure, elimination of other ailments, tests and consideration of the above symptoms. In 2004 a new test called the Snap 3DX was developed by IDEXX Laboratories in the US. The test requires only a few minutes wait for results. This test may not yet be available in Canada.

Treatment with antibiotics is often required for several weeks. Some animals may experience a "herx", a temporary worsening of symptoms, as the bacteria are killed. If laminitis is suspected, a veterinarian should be consulted to initiate preventative treatment.

Prevention of Lyme disease in horses is dependant on tick control. Daily grooming and removal of ticks is the best method of control. Tick repellants may be applied to the haircoat, especially the head, neck, legs, belly and under the tail. Use these products in spring and fall when adult ticks are most active. Ensuring pastures are reasonably short and removing brush, wood piles, etc., will decrease rodent nesting habitat, diminishing tick populations.As with dogs, when trail riding, if at all possible, try to avoid having your horse brush up against foliage on the sides of trails, thus reducing the chance of infection. Middle of the trail is best.

PART THREE

THE MEDICAL 'INTELLIGENCE' ON LYME

12

THE PROBLEM WITH
LAB TESTS!

❊ ❊ ❊

*******This next download from the Internet shows the problem with the lab tests: The complete article is worth the reading <u>especially for health care professionals!</u>

ILADS Lyme Disease Basics Page 1
Lyme Disease Basic Information
International Lyme and Associated Diseases Society (ILADS)
A Professional Research & Medical Association
PO Box 341461 · Bethesda MD 20827-1461
www.ilads.org

1. Lyme disease is prevalent across the United States. Ticks do not know geographic boundaries. A patient's county of residence does not accurately

reflect their total Lyme disease risk, since people travel, pets travel, and ticks travel. This creates a dynamic situation with many opportunities for exposure for each individual.

2. Lyme disease is a *clinical diagnosis.* Spirochetal infection of multiple organ systems causes a wide range of symptoms. Familiarity with its varied presentations is key to recognizing disseminated Lyme disease. Case reports in the medical literature document its protean manifestations.

3. *Fewer than 50%* of patients with Lyme disease recall a tick bite. In some studies this number is as low as 15% in culture proven Lyme borrelial infection.

4. *Fewer than 50%* of patients with Lyme disease recall any rash. Although the bull's eye presentation is considered classic, it is not the most common dermatologic manifestation of early-localized Lyme infection. Atypical forms of this rash are seen far more commonly. It is important to know that the Erythema Migrans rash is pathognomonic of Lyme disease and requires no further verification prior to starting 6 weeks of antibiotic therapy. Shorter treatment courses have resulted in upwards of a 40% relapse rate.

5. The CDC surveillance criteria were devised to track a narrow band of cases for epidemiologic change and were **never** set up to be used as diagnostic criteria nor were they meant to define the entire

scope of Lyme disease. This is stated in the 3/25/91 NIH report.

6. The ELISA test is unreliable, and misses 35% of culture proven Lyme (meaning only 65% sensitivity) and is unacceptable as the first step of a two step screening protocol. (By definition a screening test should have 95% sensitivity.)

7. Of patients with acute culture proven Lyme disease, *20-30%* remain seronegative *on serial Western Blot sampling.* Antibody titers also appear to decline over time; thus, the IgG Western Blot is even less sensitive in detecting chronic Lyme infection yet the IgM Western Blot may work. For "epidemiological purposes" the CDC eliminated from the Western Blot analysis the reading of bands 31 and 34. These bands are so specific to *Borrelia burgdorferi* that they have been chosen for vaccine development.

However, for patients not vaccinated for Lyme, a positive 31 or 34 band is highly indicative of *Borrelia burgdorferi* exposure.

ILADS Lyme Disease Basics Page 2

8. When used as a part of a diagnostic evaluation for Lyme disease, the Western Blot should be performed by a laboratory that reads and reports on all 16 bands as part of their routine comprehensive analysis. Laboratories (such as

SmithKline) that use FDA approved kits (for instance, Mardex's Marblot) are restricted from reporting all of the bands, as they must abide by the rules of the manufacturer. *These rules are set up in accordance with the CDC's surveillance criteria and increase the risk of false negative results.* These kits may be OK for surveillance purposes, but offer too scanty of an analysis to be useful in patient management.

9. A preponderance of evidence indicates that active ongoing spirochetal infection is the cause of the persistent symptoms in chronic Lyme disease.

10. *There has never in the history of this illness been one study that proves even in the simplest way that 30 days of antibiotic treatment cures Lyme disease.* However there is a plethora of documentation in the US and European medical literature demonstrating histologically and in culture that short courses of antibiotic treatment fail to eradicate the Lyme spirochete.

11. An uncomplicated case of chronic Lyme disease requires an average of 6-12 months of high dose antibiotic therapy. The return of symptoms and evidence of the continued presence of *Borrelia burgdorferi* indicates the need for further treatment. The very real consequences of untreated chronic persistent Lyme infection far outweigh the potential consequences of long term antibiotic therapy.

12. Many patients with Lyme disease require treatment for 1-4 years, or until the patient is symptom free. Relapses occur and maintenance antibiotics may be required.

    There are no tests available to assure us whether the organism is eradicated or the patient is cured.

13. There are 5 subspecies of *Borrelia burgdorferi, over 100 strains in the US,* and 300 strains worldwide. This diversity is thought to contribute to *Borrelia burgdorferi*'s antigenic variability and its various antibiotic resistances.

14. Antibody titers for *Babesia microti,* HGE, HME (other tick transmitted diseases)should be performed. The presence of co-infection points to probable Lyme infection, and when left untreated increases morbidity and complicates successful treatment of Lyme disease.

15. Lyme disease is the latest great imitator and should be considered in the differential diagnosis of MS, ALS, seizure and other neurologic conditions, as well as arthritis, CFS, Gulf war syndrome, ADHD, hypochondriasis, fibromyalgia, somatization disorder and patients with various difficult-to-diagnose multi-system syndromes.

See the ILADS site for updated information based on continuing research and clinical findings.

13

LYME DISEASE MEDICAL; CONTROVERSY TODAY

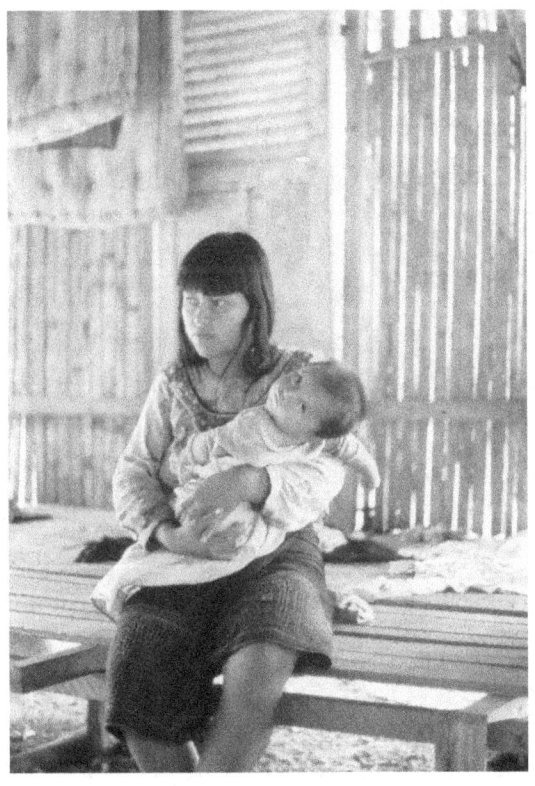

Native of Peruvian jungle with baby

⚘ ⚘ ⚘

The CDC clinical criteria for Lyme disease which exist for the purpose of monitoring the rate of Lyme disease nationally are quite narrowly defined in order to ensure a high degree of specificity in the diagnosis. These criteria are mainly useful for the early stages and rheumatological presentations of Lyme disease, such as when a patient appears with an erythema migrans rash, arthritis, a Bell's palsy, or early central neurologic Lyme disease (meningitis or encephalitis). The CDC criteria are not very helpful for helping the clinician to detect late stage neurologic Lyme disease. For example, the most common manifestation of late neurologic Lyme disease is cognitive dysfunction (often referred to as "encephalopathy"). A patient who presents with new onset encephalopathy and a positive blood test for Lyme disease would not be considered by the CDC to be a case of Lyme disease. Although the CDC recognizes that Lyme encephalopathy exists, encephalopathy is not part of the "surveillance case definition". Hence, physicians who rely on the narrow surveillance case criteria of the CDC for clinical diagnosis will fail to diagnose some patients who in fact do have Lyme disease; in these cases, the patient's treatment will either not occur or be delayed. Such delay in treatment may result in an acute treatable illness becoming a chronic less responsive one.

Other physicians who use a broader more inclusive set of clinical criteria for the diagnosis of Lyme disease will make the diagnosis of Lyme disease and initiate treatment. The latter group of doctors, by treating some patients for "probable Lyme disease", will make use of antibiotic responsiveness to confirm their diagnostic impression. These physicians, by erring on the side of not letting a patient with probable Lyme disease go untreated, will help many patients who otherwise would not get treatment; undoubtedly, however, because of the inclusiveness of their diagnostic approach, these physicians will also treat some patients with antibiotics who do not have Lyme disease. These physicians would argue that the serious consequences for physical, cognitive, and functional disability associated with chronic Lyme disease outweigh the risks of antibiotic therapy.

Both sets of doctors are practicing medicine in a reasonable fashion based on the application of certain diagnostic principles, although the therapeutic approaches differ considerably stemming from the narrow vs broad criteria for diagnosis. This is the essence of the medical controversy surrounding chronic Lyme disease. Until medical doctors have a test that definitively identifies the presence or absence of infection (and such a test does not yet exist), the controversy about the diagnosis and treatment of chronic Lyme disease will continue.

I am pleased to announce a new <u>Federal Law (Public Law 107-116)</u> that is a major benefit to the Lyme community. The bill was passed by the Senate and House and signed by President Bush on January 10, 2002. It gives the Will of Congress on issues pertaining to Lyme disease.

For over a year the LDF has worked closely with members of Congress, the Lyme Society, the Illinois and New Jersey Task Forces, physicians, and many others, on the law's tick-borne wording. We are confident it will greatly benefit physicians and patients nationwide. This is another accomplishment to help our doctors, patients, and the public.

This Public Law's Appropriations wording states that the CDC's case surveillance definition "is reportedly misused as a standard of care for healthcare reimbursement, product (test) development, medical licensing hearings, and other legal cases." This reinforces that protocols based on the case definition form inappropriate standards of care. The wording also instructs the CDC to correct this misuse! Other important wording addresses concerns over the Lyme vaccine, broadening the Lyme Case Surveillance Definition, and encouraging development of an unequivocal (perfect) test.

Karen Forschner
Lyme Disease Foundation

Here is a sample letter to send to insurance companies, licensing boards, etc.-

To Whom It May Concern: This law, signed by President Bush, reinforces that the CDC's Lyme disease (LD) Case Surveillance Definition is not valid as a standard of care for the diagnosis and treatment of Lyme disease. It also reinforces that medical protocols that use the CDC LD

Case Definition to base diagnostic and/or treatment standards misuse this protocol and are invalid. This means the Federal Government believes decisions regarding Lyme disease diagnosis, treatment and insurance reimbursement for Lyme disease care cannot be based on the CDC's Lyme disease surveillance case definition. A copy of the wording follows below.

Signed: _____

Public Law 107-116 Signed by President Bush 1/10/02 Departments of Labor, Health, and Human Services, and Education, and Related Agencies Appropriations Act 2002 This is the wording that was passed by the Senate (11/06/01, 12/20/2001) and House (10/11/01, 12/19/01) and included as part of the final bill was signed into Public Law by President George Bush on January 10, 2002. Centers for Disease Control and Prevention Lyme Disease.

"The Committee is deeply concerned about the safety of the Lyme disease vaccine (LymeRix). Over 1,000 adverse event reports were filed with the Food and Drug Administration from December 1998 to October 2000. The Committee encourages CDC to work closely with the FDA to ensure that all adverse event reports are thoroughly and expeditiously investigated to ensure public safety as the vaccine is being distributed. Investigators should pay particular attention to patients' reports of arthritis when evaluating these reports.

The Committee recognizes that the current state of laboratory testing for Lyme disease is very poor. The situation has led many people to be misdiagnosed and delayed proper treatment. The vaccine clinical trial has documented that more that one third (36 percent) of the people with Lyme disease did not test positive on the most sophisticated tests available. The ramifications of this deficit in terms of unnecessary pain, suffering and cost is staggering. The Committee directs CDC to work closely with the Food and Drug Administration to develop an unequivocal test for Lyme disease. The Committee is distressed in hearing of the widespread misuse of the current Lyme disease surveillance case definition. While the CDC does state that 'this surveillance case definition was developed for national reporting of Lyme disease: it is NOT appropriate for clinical diagnosis,' <u>the definition is reportedly misused as a standard of care for healthcare reimbursement, product (test) Development, medical licensing, and other</u> legal cases. The CDC is encouraged to aggressively pursue and correct the misuse of this definition. This includes issuing an alert to the public and physicians, as well as actively issuing letters to places misusing this definition.

The Committee recommends that the CDC strongly support the re-examination and broadening of the Lyme disease surveillance case definition by the Council of State and Territorial Epidemiologists. Voluntary and patient groups should have input into this process. Currently there is just one definition ('confirmed case') of seven possible categories. By developing other categories while leaving the current category intact, the true number of cases being diagnosed and treated will be more accurately counted, lending to improved public health planning for finding solutions to the infection. The CDC is encouraged to include a broad range of scientific viewpoints in the process of planning and executing their efforts. This means including community-based clinicians with extensive experience in treating these patients, voluntary agencies who have advocacy in their mission, and patient advocates in planning committees, meetings, and outreach efforts. National Institutes of Health - Office of the Director Lyme disease.

The Committee recommends that the NIH improve its communication across Institutes in order to better coordinate Lyme disease research and outreach to public and private scientists with the goal of stimulating research interest in this field. The Committee encourages the Office of the Director to involve NIAID, NHLBI, NINDS, NEI, NIMH, and NCCAM in promising areas of research. The Committee urges NIH officials to identify appropriate NIH advisory committees for Lyme disease representation and ensure the appointment of qualified persons. The NIH is encouraged to include a broad range of scientific viewpoints in the process of planning and executing these efforts, including community-based clinicians with extensive experience in treating these patients, voluntary agencies who have advocacy in their mission, and patient advocates. Regarding the Social Security Administration, the Committee understands that some patients with Lyme disease and other tick-borne disorders have encountered some difficulty when applying for assistance through SSA offices, due to SSA employees' unfamiliarity with these illnesses. SSA is encouraged to work on developing educational materials for SSA employees to facilitate a better understanding of the potential debilitating effects of these disorders. The Committee suggests that SSA collaborate with clinicians who have expertise on the multi-system chronic effects of Lyme, as well as patient and voluntary communities, to accomplish this goal."

14

MEDICAL ABSTRACTS AND OTHER INFORMATION THAT WILL HELP YOU IN YOUR OWN RESEARCH EFFORTS

❃ ❃ ❃

Here is very interesting story of a physician who was diagnosed with ALS which paralyzes a victim from the lower extremeties all the way to the upper body and death occurs within approximately 5 years !

ILADS WELCOMES PHYSICIAN RECOVERING FROM ALS DOCTOR'S CASE SUPPORTS THEORY LYME DISEASE MAY BE THE CAUSE OF ALS

Bethesda, MD. September 2, 2004 - The International Lyme and Associated Diseases Society (ILADS) strengthened its impressive membership today with the addition of

Dr. Dave Martz of Colorado Springs, who joined ILADS 15 months after being diagnosed with Amyotrophic Lateral Sclerosis (ALS). In April of 2003, Dr. Martz began suffering weakness and pain in his muscles. Dr. Martz soon lost much of his mobility. His condition worsened forcing him to retire from the medical practice he loves.

After six frustrating months with hope fading, Dr. Martz discovered the work of Dr. Gregory Bach of Colmar, Pennsylvania. Dr. Bach, who is a member of ILADS, suggested a link between ALS and Lyme disease. IGeneX Reference Laboratory of Palo Alto then confirmed Lyme bacteria in Dr. Martz. Dr. Martz then sought out a local ILADS physician who started Lyme disease treatment based on the recommendations of Dr. Bach. The results were dramatic.

"Before I found Lyme "literate" professionals, I could only function at a level of about 20 percent," says Dr. Martz. "But now that I'm in expert hands, I am up to 75 percent of full function and I hope to return to work soon as a physician, helping others with Chronic Lyme disease." An Internist, and past president of the Colorado Medical Society, he is committed to giving others opportunities that have been given to him.

The Center for Disease Control says that Lyme disease may be under-reported by as much as ten-fold. This means as many as a quarter of a million Americans may contract Lyme disease each year, yet most of them are unaware of it.

ILADS president, Dr. Steven Phillips, says, "Dr. Martz is an example of the many physicians and medical experts we encourage to join ILADS so we can continue to raise awareness and make vital advances in the world-wide fight against Lyme disease."

For more information about Lyme disease go to www.ilads.org CONTACT:

Barbara Buchman (301) 263-1080

Christi O'Connor (415) 883-2491

Intermediate uveitis and Lyme borreliosis.

Breeveld J, Rothova A, Kuiper H.
Department of Ophthalmology, Academic Medical Centre, Amsterdam, The Netherlands.

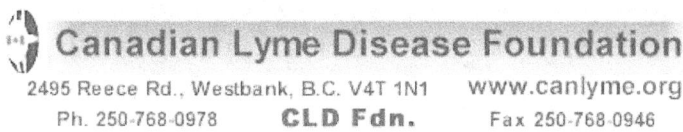

Canadian Lyme Disease Foundation
2495 Reece Rd., Westbank, B.C. V4T 1N1 www.canlyme.org
Ph. 250-768-0978 **CLD Fdn.** Fax 250-768-0946

A case of chronic intermediate uveitis and associated classic snowbanking (pars planitis) with severe cystoid macular edema probably due to Lyme borreliosis is reported. Despite a disease duration of 10 years the patient's ocular symptoms and visual acuity responded promptly to intravenous ceftriaxone treatment. This case demonstrates that periodic reevaluation of patients with intermediate uveitis is necessary to obtain a specific diagnosis which may include Lyme borreliosis.

The etiology of uveitis: the role of infections with special reference to Lyme borreliosis.

Mikkila H, Seppala I, Leirisalo-Repo M, Immonen I, Karma A.

Department of Ophthalmology, University of Helsinki, Finland.

PURPOSE: To assess the distribution of different uveitis entities and to evaluate their associations with infections, especially Lyme borreliosis. METHODS: During a one-year period 160 consecutive uveitis patients were evaluated in a university clinic. Selected tests were performed depending on the medical history of the patient and the clinical picture of the ocular inflammation. RESULTS: Uveitis was classified into selected entities for 74.4% of the patients. A direct infection was suggested to be linked with uveitis in 23 patients (14.4%). Lyme borreliosis, toxoplasmosis, and herpetic infections were the most frequently seen, in seven patients (4.3%) each. All patients with Lyme uveitis had manifestations of the posterior segment of the eye, such as vitritis, retinal vasculitis, neuroretinitis, chorioretinitis, or optic neuropathy. CONCLUSION: Infections are an important cause of uveitis in a university clinic. Lyme borreliosis is a newly recognised uveitis entity which should be kept in mind in the differential diagnosis of intermediate or posterior uveitis in areas endemic for Lyme borreliosis.

Identity Theft!

Acta Neurol Scand. 2006 Apr;113(4):248–55

Microbes in tissues living under the Alzheimer Name – Identity Theft?

Herein, we submit a case study which offers a new cognitive model for Alzheimer's disease. It is unknown how many persons might fit into this model, but if even one person could potentially benefit, we believe that it is in the public interest to discuss the case of Mr Paul Christensen. http://www.canlyme.com/alan_alzheimers_case_study_2006.html

The above web page gives a clear indication that Alzheimer's disease is related to Lyme spirochetal infection!

FDA Chief found Guilty !

From http://www.signonsandiego.com/news/nation/20061016-1324-fda-crawford.html
By Pete Yost

ASSOCIATED PRESS
1:24 p.m. October 16, 2006
Ex-FDA chief expected to plead guilty in conflict of interest case

WASHINGTON – Former FDA chief Lester Crawford has agreed to plead guilty to charges of failing to disclose a financial interest in PepsiCo Inc. and other firms regulated by his agency, his lawyer said Monday.

The Justice Department accused the former head of the Food and Drug Administration in court papers of falsely reporting that he had sold stock in companies when he continued holding shares in the firms governed by FDA rules.

Court papers say Crawford chaired the Food and Drug Administration's Obesity Working Group while he and his wife owned shares worth at least $62,000 in soft drink and snack food manufacturer Pepsico Inc., based in Purchase, N.Y. In addition, the documents say, he held stock worth at least $78,000 in food product manufacturer Sysco Corp., based in Houston.

While he and his wife owned the stock, the panel Crawford chaired met with representatives from the packaged food industry and gave congressional testimony encouraging manufacturers to relabel serving sizes to give calorie counts greater prominence.

Crawford "is going to plead guilty to two misdemeanors tomorrow afternoon and he is going to admit his financial disclosures had errors and omissions, mostly with his wife's continued ownership of stocks," said Crawford's lawyer, Barbara Van Gelder.

"At the end of the day, he owned these stocks and he will admit he owned them while he was at the FDA and he will take responsibility for that," said Van Gelder. She said Crawford was not disputing the government's claims in what she called a plea agreement.

Accused of making a false writing and conflict of interest, Crawford was scheduled to appear before a federal magistrate Tuesday afternoon. Each charge carries a maximum penalty of one year in prison.

The papers say Crawford failed to disclose his income from exercising stock options in Embrex Inc. of Research Triangle Park, N.C., an agriculture biotechnology company that has been regulated by FDA. Crawford had been a member of Embrex's board of directors, according to federal filings.

Crawford, a veterinarian, abruptly resigned from the FDA in September 2005 but gave no reason for his departure. He had held the top position for just two months but had been acting head of the agency for more than a year.

According to the Justice Department's court papers:

- A government ethics official inquired about Crawford's ownership of stock in several companies FDA regulates and Crawford replied in a Dec. 28, 2004, e-mail that "Sysco and Kimberly-Clark have in fact been sold." Actually, the court papers state, Crawford knew that he or his wife still held shares in both.

- Even though financial reporting requirements for federal officials say all income must be disclosed, Crawford failed to reveal $8,000 in income from the exercise of Embrex stock options in 2003, and failed to report $20,000 from the sale of Embrex stock options in 2004.

To add to the problem above here is an excerpt from a major story from Reader's Digest – April 4th, 2008. The title is "Strong Medicine"

"Recent headlines have uncovered one shocking lapse after another at the Food and Drug Administration. A popular diabetes drug can sharply increase the risk of heart attack, a finding the agency knew but took two years to reveal . An FDA approved antibiotic can destroy your liver in just five days. And despite mounting concerns about the safety of Chinese-made drugs, the agency had only enough field inspectors last year to check a mere 13 of the 714 Chinese factories that produce medicines for U.S. consumers. Many of the nation's leading doctors, scientists, and lawmakers now agree that the FDA is in crisis...." Apparently, the organization is underfunded, understaffed and absolutely dysfunctional !"

"Think your pacemaker, heart valve, microwave oven or morning vitamin was inspected?" asks former associate commissioner William Hubbard. "Dream on." A chilling new report commissioned by the FDA's advisory Science Board describes an organization nearly out of control".... You the reader of this book might want to get a copy of the article from Reader's Digest.!

Birds, Birds, Birds~ what are they doing?!

Contact: John D. Scott,
President, Lyme Disease Association of Ontario
519-843-3646 (9:00–11:30 a.m., 2:00–4:30 p.m.)
jnkscott@freespace.net

Muhammad G. Morshed, Ph.D.,
Head, Zoonotic and Emerging Pathogens, Laboratory Services,
British Columbia Centre for Disease Control,
604-660-6074
mmorshed@interchange.ubc.ca

Mystery behind the spread of Lyme in Canada Uncovered by Canadian Researchers

Startling new study has unlocked the mystery surrounding growing infections of Lyme disease in parts of Canada where disease-carrying ticks are not native to the area, and offering doctors an explanation for the appearance of Lyme-related symptoms among their patients.

Lyme disease advocates want Canadian doctors to understand this now because October is the peak month for black-legged tick adults, a time when hunters and hikers are out in the bush and vulnerable to infection.

It turns out the guilty culprits are the billions of songbirds that migrate into and out of Canada every year.

These findings are critical, say Lyme disease advocates, because they will finally offer an explanation to doctors who insist that their patients cannot have contracted Lyme disease because the ticks that carry it aren't native to the area. The study points the finger squarely at birds wintering in southern climates and can carry tick species 5000 km during their northern flight to Canada every spring. The study, led by Prof. Muhammad G. Morshed, the head of Zoonotic and Emerging Pathogens at the British Columbia Centre for Disease Control, recently published its findings in the

Journal of Parasitology. Advocates for greater awareness of Lyme Disease in Canada say that until now, many patients were routinely told by their doctors that they do not have the disease because the ticks that carry the illness and its co-infections were not native to their area.

This has led to a rash of misdiagnoses for MS, Parkinsons, Lupus, fibromyalgia, Reynaud's, various forms of arthritis, and even Lou Gehrig's Disease, they add.

"This has frustrated many patients who eventually get in touch with our association," said John Scott, president and co-founder with his wife, Kit, of the Ontario Lyme Disease Association.

"Based on this belief, doctors refuse to test patients for Lyme or even consider it as a diagnosis because the disease vectors are not thought to be in the area, and nobody is telling the doctors any differently."

Scott notes that patients end up travelling to the United States for diagnosis, or to major urban areas like Toronto and Vancouver to find the few Canadian doctors with any experience treating and diagnosing the disease which can attack any organ in the body and affect the central nervous system.

A recent spate of feature articles in daily newspapers in Halifax, Ottawa, Peterborough and in the Globe and Mail have highlighted the frustration Canadian Lyme patients experience in their efforts to get a diagnosis and decent treatment in Canada.

The link to songbirds is significant because studies show that billions of birds migrate into and out of Canada each year playing an important role in the dispersal of ticks infected with the Lyme disease spirochete.

Biology researchers know that ground-dwelling songbirds, which forage among leaf litter and low-lying vegetation, are particularly susceptible to tick attachment.

"In essence," said Scott, "the ticks hitch a ride and get carried to Canada, where they drop off, attach to people and make them sick."

Researchers studied 25 sites across Canada and collected nine different tick species from 32 species of birds. In eastern Canada blacklegged ticks, Ioxdes scapularis, or "deer ticks" were removed from spring migratory birds.

Birds carry bacteria across the hemispheres: Migratory birds transmit borreliosis

May 20, 2005

Migrating birds transmit different forms of the Borrelia bacterium or Borrelia spirochetes to every corner of the globe. Birds are especially prone to Borrelia infected ticks during their autumn and spring migrations. The bacteria may also persist for several months in the birds and it may then be reactivated in response to migration. Borrelia spirochetes and the role of birds as global transmitters of the bacteria have been investigated by a Swedish research group led by Professor Sven Bergström. The group is part of a Finnish-Swedish research consortium included in the Microbes and Man Research Programme, which is co-funded by the Academy of Finland and the Swedish Foundation for Strategic Research.

Migratory birds play an important role in the transmission of Lyme borreliosis. The fact that the same type of Lyme disease exists in both the northern and the southern hemisphere shows that birds participate in the natural circulation of Borrelia spirochetes by carrying them all across the globe.

Previously, it was thought that only mammals could function as reservoir hosts for Borrelia infected ticks. The research results of the Bergström group show that Borrelia infected ticks can exist in birds, as well - i.e. without a mammal reservoir.

Lyme Borreliosis is an infectious disease caused by the Borrelia bacterium. It can cause eczemas, arthritis and, at the worst, even different kinds of neurological disorders. In Finland, a couple of thousand people are infected by the disease each year.

Microbes and Man Research Programme is a three-year programme during 2003-2005. With the budget of 5,4 million euros 15 projects are funded. The programme is implemented in Finnish-Swedish collaboration.

Suomen Akatemia (Academy of Finland)

<u>Is this the only way our medical professionals will start thinking "outside the medical box?"</u>

From the <u>Cecil Whig</u> newspaper (1999)

Jury awards $1.7 million to Cecil teen
By Carl Hamilton, Whig Staff Writer (Maryland, USA)

ELKTON - A civil jury awarded more than $1.7 million Monday to a Port Deposit teen who suffers long-term health problems because local physicians failed to diagnose his Lyme disease. This is believed to be the highest award of damages in Cecil County history, according to veteran lawyers and court officials.

The six-member jury deliberated nearly eight hours before concluding that Chesapeake Family Practice Group on High Street in Elkton breached the standard of medical care when treating Aaron Murray. That breach, according to the jury, directly resulted in Murray's physical problems, including his IQ reportedly dropping as much as 29 points.

Int J Dermatol. 2006 Sep;45(9):1104-6.

Treatment of lichen sclerosus with antibiotics
* Shelley WB, * Shelley ED, * Amurao CV.

From the Division of Dermatology, Department of Medicine, Medical University of Ohio, Ohio, OH.

Current therapy for lichen sclerosus centers on topical steroids, particularly clobetasol propionate. As some evidence suggests an infectious etiology owing to Borrelia, we studied the effect of penicillin and cephalosporin therapy on patients with lichen sclerosus who had responded poorly to treatment with potent topical corticosteroids.

Fifteen patients with lichen sclerosus were treated for 3-21 months with either penicillin or cephalosporins in an observational study. Thirteen patients (nine women, four men) received penicillin, including intramuscular penicillin G benzathine suspension and/or oral penicillin V potassium, amoxicillin, or amoxicillin/clavulanate potassium. Two additional men received cephalosporins, either intramuscular ceftriaxone sodium or oral cefadroxil monohydrate.

All patients showed a significant response, evident within a few weeks. Most striking was the rapid relief of pain, pruritus and burning. Four patients cleared completely, four experienced marked improvement, and the remaining seven had a favorable improvement of symptoms with incomplete clearing of lesions.

We recommend treatment of lichen sclerosus with either intramuscular ceftriaxone every 3 weeks or intramuscular penicillin every 2-3 weeks. The addition of oral penicillin or cephalosporin presumably helps maintain antibiotic blood levels and may be a sufficient treatment in some cases.

[Note: The above skin disease creates moderate to severe itching especially in the scalp occipital areas. Scratching the skin tends to cause scales and plaques on the skin area involved].

Fever Improves Autism Symptoms

Reason for Improvement Not Understood

By Salynn Boyles
WebMD Medical News

Reviewed by Louise Chang, MD

Dec. 3, 2007 – Children with autism appear to improve when they have a fever, according to intriguing new research that could lead to a better understanding of the disorder.

Fever was associated with less hyperactivity, improved communication, and less irritability in the study involving children with autism and related disorders.

Anecdotal reports of improvements in autism symptoms related to fever have circulated for years, but the research represents the first scientific investigation into the observed association.

While kids with autism might be expected to be calmer and less hyperactive when they have fevers, the improvement in communication and socialization seen in the study suggests that fever directly affects brain function, pediatric neurologist Andrew Zimmerman, MD, of Baltimore's Kennedy Krieger Institute, tells WebMD.

"The improvement in symptoms may mean the underlying wiring of the brain (of an autistic child) develops more normally than we have thought," he says, adding that the problem may lie with the connections within the brain responsible for sending information.

"Somehow fever appears to be changing the ability to make these connections," he says.

4 out of 5 Kids With Fever Improved

The study involved 30 children with autism spectrum disorders, including autism, who were observed by parents during and immediately after experiencing a fever of 100.4 degrees or greater, and seven days after being without fever.

The parents were asked to complete standardized behavior questionnaires during the three time points designed to assess behavior. Parents of children with autism spectrum disorders who did not experience fever were also surveyed at related time points.

More than 80% of the children with fever in the study showed some improvement in behavior during temperature elevations, the researchers reported in the December issue of the journal *Pediatrics.*

Further analysis showed that behavior improvement was not dependent on the degree of fever.

Zimmerman and lead researcher Laura K. Curran, PhD, tell WebMD that more study is needed to confirm the findings.

"We'd like to interview more families to better understand this," Zimmerman says. "And at the chemical level, we'd like to have blood samples from children while they have fever to analyze what is going on."

Autism, Fever, and Cytokines

One theory is that fever may affect brain function at the cellular level by influencing the production of immune-system signaling proteins known as cytokines.

If this proves to be the case, the finding could result in treatments for autism spectrum disorders that target cytokine expression.

"That would be a long way off, but it is certainly within the realm of possibility," Zimmerman says.

Marguerite Kirst Colston says the new research is significant because it is one of the first to examine the symptoms parents deal with in biological terms.

Colston is a spokeswoman for the American Society of Autism (ASA) and the mother of a 7-year-old son with autism.

"We are hearing more and more about this from parents," she tells WebMD. "Children seem calmer when they are sick and they seem to tolerate closeness and touch better. We have all sort of marveled at this."

Colston hopes the research will lead to more studies that look beyond the genetics of autism.

"The more we study what happens biologically, as well as genetically, the more insight we may have into how to treat children to improve their symptoms," she says. "I would like to see us focus on questions like, 'What helps these kids learn?' and 'What makes them feel better?' 'What do people with autism need to live well?' I'm a parent who has tried a lot of things, and I have no idea."

Heat Shock Proteins: Basics
http://www.antigenics.com/products/tech/hsp/

basics | in-depth information | how they work: animation| applications | reclinical studies | references

What are heat shock proteins and how do they work?

Heat shock proteins (HSPs), also called stress proteins, are a group of proteins that are present in all cells in all life forms. They are induced when a cell undergoes various types of environmental stresses like heat, cold and oxygen deprivation.

Heat shock proteins are also present in cells under perfectly normal conditions. They act like 'chaperones,' making sure that the cell's proteins are in the right shape and in the right place at the right time. For example, HSPs help new or distorted proteins fold into shape, which is essential for their function. They also shuttle proteins from one compartment to another inside the cell, and transport old proteins to 'garbage disposals' inside the cell. Heat shock proteins are also believed to play a role in the presentation of pieces of proteins (or peptides) on the cell surface to help the immune system recognize diseased cells.

What do heat shock proteins have to do with cancer?

For decades it has been known that animals can be 'vaccinated' against cancer. This is how it works: Tumor cells can be weakened, or *attenuated*, and injected like a vaccine into a mouse. Afterwards, if these same tumor cells, at full strength, are injected into the mouse, the mouse will reject the tumor cells and cancer will not develop. However, if a mouse has not been vaccinated in this manner, the tumor cells will 'take' and the mouse will develop cancer.

Although it was clear that animals could be vaccinated against cancer, for a long time it was not known how it worked. Then about 25 years ago, a graduate student named Pramod Srivastava began a series of experiments. He took tumor cells, broke them open, and separated the different parts of the cells into fractions. He then used each of the fractions as 'vaccines' to see which fraction protected the mice from developing cancer. After many experiments, he found that the element responsible for protecting the mice was heat shock proteins. [More]

How are heat shock proteins involved in generating immune response?

Heat shock proteins trigger immune response through activities that occur both inside the cell (intracellular) and outside the cell (extracellular).

Intracellular activities

Because of the normal functions of heat shock proteins inside the cell (such as helping proteins fold, preparing proteins for disposal, etc.), HSPs end up binding virtually every protein made within the cell. This means that at any given time, HSPs can be found inside the cell bound to a wide array of peptides that represent a 'library' of all the proteins inside the cell. This library contains normal peptides that are found in all cells as well as abnormal peptides that are only found in sick cells.

Research suggests that inside the cell, heat shock proteins take the peptides and hand them over to another group of <u>molecules</u>. These other molecules take the abnormal peptides that are found only in sick cells and move them from inside the cell to outside on the cell's surface. When the abnormal peptides are displayed in this way, they act as red flags, warning the <u>immune system</u> that the cell has become sick. These abnormal peptides are called antigens — a term that describes any substance capable of triggering an <u>immune response</u>.

Extracellular activities

Heat shock proteins are normally found inside cells. When they are found outside the cell, it indicates that a cell has become so sick that it has died and spilled out all of its contents. This kind of messy, unplanned death is called necrosis, and only occurs when something is very wrong with the cell. Extracellular HSPs are one of the most powerful ways of sending a 'danger signal' to the immune system in order to generate a response that can help to get rid of an infection or disease. [More]

How does Antigenics' heat shock protein technology work?

Antigenics' heat shock protein technology works by mimicking the 'danger signal' believed to be naturally triggered by <u>extracellular</u> HSPs. Depending on the abnormal <u>peptides</u> contained within the HSP-associated 'library' of proteins that have spilled out of the cell, the immune system can be activated to target different cancers and certain infectious agents.

Antigenics' investigational patient-specific cancer vaccine Oncophage (vitespen; formerly HSPPC-96) consists of HSP-peptide complexes that have been isolated from individual patient's cancer cells. Because cancer is so incredibly variable, the abnormal peptides found within diseased cells are different from cancer to cancer and from person to person. Therefore, this library of abnormal peptides is unique to each individual's disease and can be thought of as the cancer's 'fingerprint.'

When the vaccine is injected into the body, the fingerprint of HSP-peptide complexes can directly encounter the immune system's cells, which is designed to stimulate the immune cells to target cancer cells bearing this fingerprint.

Author's comments:

Could this be a partial answer to the questions of what happens when the body temperature becomes a fever?

In the case of Autism, fever which raises the core body temperature seems to help increase certain chemicals in the body which allows better cerebration and as result better communication and normal emotional behavior in patients with Autism.

Again, I have a number of friends and others who have used the hot tub technique to raise their body temperature "because it feels good after the treatment". A number of these suffer from the effects of Lyme disease which makes their joints and muscles ache as well as disturbs their sleep and normal mental and emotional ttranquility. They are very satisfied that the heat is not only relaxing, but also "healing" them ! There should be a study done on this modality of "hydro-thermia" which would be cheaper and less damaging than everything else we have tried and still use! Finally, let me tell you about <u>Stan</u> who at 50 years of age was diagnosed with Parkinson's disease. He also had Bell's Palsy for 13 years. His doctor was unable to help him or his wife who was wearing herself out trying to take care of her invalid husband. Some family members who lived in another State decided to encourage Stan to go to a Health Institute in one of the Southern States of America. This clinic specializes in Natural Remedies including hydro-therapy like Russian steam baths and hot tub soaks which could raise the core body temperature to 103-104 degrees F. The food is provided (Vegan in general) and no medications are administered (except that which the patient brings from his physician)!

With his wife accompanying him, Stan travelled from Texas to Alabama via Atlanta on Delta airlines though wheelchair bound. He had turned 65 years of age and had almost lost all hope of ever being well again...

Within a couple of weeks of treatment Stan was vastly improved and by the sixth week, he was able to walk 1-3 miles daily and also do some bicycle exercises. He has returned home and is now living a reasonably normal life.

His wife has made arrangements to have Stan's treatment program continued at the home base and is extremely happy to see how vastly improved her husband is today! His doctor (with some prodding) had Stan's blood drawn before he left for his treatment in Alabama. Before the patient returned home the results of the blood work done at IgeneX (specializing in tick borne diseases) in Palo Alto, CA) showed that *Stan was infected with Lyme disease!* Now we are beginning to see the connection between many neurological syndromes caused by tick borne infections. And maybe getting a peek at a pre-emptive plan to win the battle of Lyme and all its co-infections!?

Is your teenager with Lyme disease struggling in school?

WILTON, CT - October 13, 2005 - Have you watched with sadness and frustration as your teen's academic skills have declined since he developed Lyme disease? Does she forget the simplest assignments or seem unable to stay organized? Does he stumble over tasks he used to perform with ease?

Patrick McAuliffe, M.Ed.-a doctoral candidate at Teacher's College, is recruiting teenagers for a study on the relationship between Lyme disease and cognition. As a school psychologist in Ridgefield, Connecticut, and as a facilitator of the Wilton Lyme Disease Support Group for Teens, Mr. McAuliffe has extensive experience with emotionally fragile teens in general and Lyme disease patients in particular.

Lyme disease may have a dramatic, disruptive effect on teens trying to meet the academic and emotional challenges they encounter every day. Some students become so ill they can't attend school on a daily basis. Those who make it to class may struggle with debilitating symptoms such as fatigue, headaches and joint pain. They may also experience a sharp, sudden decline in academic achievement. Teens with Lyme may well be overwhelmed as they try to meet the intense academic and social pressures of teenage life.

Mr. McAuliffe is conducting the first research project to examine the cognitive effects of Lyme disease in adolescents. The need is great, since Lyme is a controversial disease and spreading rapidly. Estimated to affect as many as 54 % of households in some communities, Lyme disease case reports doubled from 1991 to 2000, and have since risen a dramatic 40% between 2001 and 2002. Children are at special risk, since they spend so much time outdoors in their yards or on school grounds.

Objective research with appropriate psychological instruments is vitally important in order to properly evaluate teens suffering with Lyme. If Lyme's cognitive consequences are not identified and treated, the results can be devastating, leading to school difficulty and even school failure. The social consequences can also be extremely painful.

About the Study

Adolescents in high school between the ages of 13 and 18, both with and without Lyme disease, are eligible to participate. Parents will be screened by phone about their teen's medical history. If eligible, the teen will be given various psychological tests that measure cognitive functioning. Teens and parents will learn the results of the tests, which will provide helpful insights into their issues and needs.

Participants will also receive a $20.00 gift certificate to Amazon.com.

About the researcher, Patrick McAuliffe, M.Ed.

Patrick McAuliffe, M.Ed. is a doctoral candidate in the school psychology program at Teacher's College, specializing in Neurosciences and Education.

In that capacity, he has trained at a hospital-based neuropsychological assessment service, a residential treatment facility for children and adolescents, a school-based health clinic, and in the public schools.

Mr. McAuliffe is currently a school psychologist in Ridgefield, Connecticut. He designed and runs an in-school therapeutic program for emotionally fragile high school students.

Before graduate school, Mr. McAuliffe worked as an evaluator with Dr. Brian Fallon of Columbia University on a pioneering study regarding neuropsychiatric Lyme disease in children and adolescents. Dr. Fallon is an advisor on Mr. McAuliffe's current research project.

About the Lyme Disease Support Groups

The Wilton Lyme Disease Support Group for Adults was established in 1998 to provide information and support to patients and families coping with Lyme disease. Teenagers were offered a group of their own in 2001.

Well over 600 patients have now utilized the groups' services, which include professionally facilitated monthly meetings and periodic educational events.

Teens meet the first Tuesday of every month at 4:30 PM. Young people struggling with Lyme find support, hope and the opportunity to befriend peers facing similar challenges. Patrick McAuliffe, M.Ed., a school psychologist, offers specific social and academic coping strategies.

Adults meet the second Wednesday of every month at 7:30 PM. Lyme patients, together with family and friends, share information and support on a variety of topics. Subjects range from the disease itself, to navigating the healthcare system, to coping with chronic illness at work or in relationships. The group has been facilitated since its inception by clinical psychologist Douglas Bunnell, Ph.D.

The groups are co-facilitated by Master's candidate Yvonne Bokhour. She and Jay Lux, a nurse with a master's in public health, also handle the groups' administration, which include regular educational events.

For more information about Mr. McAuliffe's research study, please visit or write Pmcauliffe@lymediseaseresearch.com.

To learn more about the Wilton Lyme Disease Support Groups, which meet at Comstock Community Center in Wilton, call Yvonne at 203 594 9077 or write kos1@earthlink.net. The Washingtonian Jan. 1991

*************This is an excellent story of how Lyme can affect certain people. Go to the web page below and read the entire 7 pages approx. Extremely valuable especially for Pediatricians and Neurologists!*

Medicine by Neil Raven—http://www.canlyme.com/bike.html

Title: <u>Bicycle Boy</u>

his Behavior was Compulsive: It's Orogins Unknown; then a good doctor finally figured it out and a miracle happened!

He was 12 years old, and every day he pedalled furiously on his stationary bicycle for as many hours as they would allow him. He was so absorbed in his effort that it was all they could do to get him to stop for meals........[get the rest of the story from the above web site!]

<u>Historic Move by CT Attorney General to Investigate IDSA Guidelines Process Gives Hope to Thousands of Lyme Disease Patients</u>

Statement from Pat Smith, President, Lyme Disease Association

HARTFORD, Conn.—(BUSINESS WIRE)—The national non-profit Lyme Disease Association (LDA), representing more Lyme disease patients than any organization in the United States, applauds Connecticut

State Attorney General Richard Blumenthal for beginning an investigation into the Infectious Diseases Society of America (IDSA) Lyme disease guidelines development process. In an unprecedented move, the Attorney General's office filed a Civil Investigative Demand (CID) to look into possible anti-trust violations by the IDSA in connection with exclusionary conduct and monopolization in the development of the Lyme guidelines.

Although unprecedented, the LDA feels this action is vitally necessary to protect the welfare of chronic Lyme patients nationwide whose treatments have been impacted by the stance taken by the IDSA. Their guidelines deny the existence of chronic infectious Lyme disease and list as "not recommended" most of the conventional medical treatments prescribed by physicians as well as alternative treatments often chosen by patients for any Lyme manifestation. Even some nutritional supplements should not be an option according to IDSA.

Clinical guidelines now drive the standard of care, and these IDSA guidelines have already been published on the CDC website. They are being used to deny treatment reimbursement and will have a continued chilling effect on the small numbers of treating physicians, since clinical discretion is not recommended in the guidelines.

The October 2006 guidelines do not acknowledge that a complex bacterium such as the Lyme disease spirochete could possibly survive in the body and the brain, evading the immune system and short-term courses of antibiotics, nor do they take into consideration any other professional diagnostic or treatment guidelines such as those published by the International Lyme and Associated Diseases Society (ILADS), which discuss chronic disease diagnostic and treatment modalities. The IDSA also refused to allow patient or chronic disease-treating physician input into the guidelines process through the LDA and ILADS, respectively, although both organizations requested to be a part of the process.

The national LDA and its affiliates Time for Lyme (CT) and the California Lyme Disease Association and ILADS, a professional medical organization, had appealed to the Attorney General on behalf of patients and treating physicians. We are encouraged by the issuance of the CID, and we hope that this will lead to actions that will guarantee patients the right to be treated and support physicians' right to treat using clinical discretion.

Letter to the Editor-Clinical Infectious Diseases
Dec. 15th, 2006
Re: Infectious Disease Society of America; Lyme Disease
   Clinical Practice Guidelines
From: J.M. Wilson, President, Canadian Lyme Disease
   Foundation,   250-768-0978,   jimwilson@telus.net
   www.canlyme.com

The Canadian Lyme Disease Foundation has several concerns with the guidelines.

I shall elaborate.

Erythema Migrans rash

Throughout the document, the erythema migrans rash (EM) is referred to 108 times and is claimed to be the predominant diagnostic feature of LD. Headaches, fatigue, cognitive dysfunction, neuropsychiatric issues, myalgias, tremors, tics and parasthesias are given little or no attention, yet they can present in all stages of the illness; the EM rash, on the other hand, normally does not, and has been overemphasized as a predominant indicator of the disease [1]. As reported by Dr. S. Banerjee in 1995, for example, only 18% of confirmed cases reported a rash [2]. The research studies cited in the guidelines in support of percentages relative to rash incidence were not designed specifically to measure incidence of the EM rash therefore minimal value can be given to the data.

Symptomatic Chronic LD and Late Stage LD

The following quote from the guidelines is evidence of poor scholarship; "There is no convincing biologic evidence for the existence of symptomatic chronic *B. burgdorferi* infection among patients after receipt of recommended treatment regimens for LD." Strong evidence exists to the contrary in both animal and human model studies, and has for years [3].

Late stage LD is very poorly defined. Arthritic and neurologic manifestations are discussed, but are not well linked to the various symptoms that coexist with them. It is this array of variable symptoms, many times in the absence of arthritis or classic neurological manifestations, that collectively are so disabling in terms of quality of life for the patient and costly for governments in terms of disability payments. The guideline refers to many of these symptoms as "aches and pains of daily living" yet no research has been presented that has had the specific design of determining all the symptoms of late LD. Symptoms such as overwhelming fatigue, pain, muscle dysfunction, cognitive dysfunction, psychiatric issues, breathing restrictions, eyesight and hearing problems, bowel dysfunction and other manifestations that can be objectively measured, if proper measuring tools are employed, are common to late LD. Labelling these as "aches and pains of daily living" or as a "post-lyme disease syndrome" is a travesty at worst and premature at best. Many symptoms have been discounted. In the guidelines, entire classes of potential therapies are discounted because of this poor recognition of symptoms.

Seronegative Lyme Disease

In Grignolo, et al, 50% of PCR positive results of serum and cerebrospinal fluid samples corresponded to patients who were true positives at clinical examination but negatives at serologic tests. Over 60% of positive urine samples belonged to patients who had negative serologic results from analysis of serum [4]. In many other studies seronegative LD was proven [5].

In light of the above, and of the large global databank of LD research, until a definitive diagnostic test is found few conclusions can be drawn about late stage LD. The often referred to 'two-tiered testing' is not accurate enough to identify LD reliably [5,6]. In addition, until a comprehensive series of post-mortem studies of many similarly presenting diagnoses (e.g. Multiple Sclerosis, Alzheimer's, Chronic Fatigue Syndrome, etc.) is conducted to look for evidence of spirochaetal infection, few conclusions can be drawn about what objective symptoms are to be attributed to late LD.

The IDSA guidelines are far too exclusive, and thus inadequate, as a health care guide for physicians. The document represents a small cohort of authors largely supporting each others work. The guidelines do not meet the stated objective of the guidelines document itself.

The IDSA guidelines should be withdrawn and replaced with a document written in collaboration with victim groups and treating physicians.

1. Stricker RB, Lautin A, and Burrascano JJ. 2006. LD: The Quest for Magic Bullets. *Chemotherapy*. 52: 53–59.
2. Gill R., Banerjee S. and Banerjee M. 1995. LD Cases Acquired in British Columbia 1992-1994 *canlyme.com/vanc1995.html*
3. http://www.lymeinfo.net/medical/LDPersist.pdf
4. Grignolo MC, Buffrini L, Monteforte P, Rovetta G. 2001 Reliability of a polymerase chain reaction (PCR) technique in the diagnosis of Lyme borreliosis. *Minerva Med*. 2001 92: 29-33.
5. http://www.lymeinfo.net/medical/LDSeronegativity.pdf

6. Coulter P, Lema C, Flayhart D, Linhardt AS, Aucott JN, Auwaeter PG, Dumler JS. 2005. Two-Year Evaluation of *Borrelia burgdorferi* Culture and Supplemental Tests for Definitive Diagnosis of Lyme Disease. *J. Clin. Microbiol.* 43: 5080-5084.

Here is a link where you can find Lyme disease in most countries of the world:

http://www.geocities.com/HotSprings/Oasis/6455/international-links.html

International Links on Lyme Disease

Lyme disease is a serious bacterial infection caused by a tick bite and affects humans and animals.

Links on this page labeled "MEDLINE" are links to citations of medical and scientific articles from the National Institutes of Health (NIH), National Library of Medicine (NLM)

• *This is one of the best reports I've seen on how MS and Lyme disease are geostatistically related! Excellent job!*

A Geostatistical Analysis of Possible Spirochetal Involvement in Multiple Sclerosis and Other Related Diseases

http://www.canlyme.com/megan_geostatistical_analysis2.html

15

CONCLUSION

✻ ✻ ✻

A final word from the front lines

There isn't a Lyme-infected tick hidden behind every bush! Lyme disease hasn't become a national horror story. Not yet…For some, however, it is already a horror story! I believe the more we understand this elusive disease, the better we can relate to others who may be suffering many of the symptoms that plague hundreds of thousands and perhaps millions of persons worldwide – the work of this often mis-diagnosed "terrorist bacterium." When I first came face to face with the Lyme terrorist I didn't know what I was up against. Early symptoms can be misleadingly commonplace: stiff finger joints, flu-like symptoms, insomnia.

Then came the succession of symptoms that couldn't be ignored or set aside: Tired, listless feelings that wouldn't go away, tingling toes and fingers with pin pricking pains anywhere and everywhere whenever the bacterium decided to strike again.

My medical ignorance regarding the Lyme terrorist finally pushed me to seek the clues I needed to fight this "devilish" thing that tormented me for months on end; reappearing as different symptoms. Extreme itchy scalp, and strange skin lesions...then hip pain followed by neck pain with spasm and low back ache which never seemed to let up! Headaches which made even my eyeballs ache! A litany of symptoms which would take more than a page or two to list!

It's said that "there is great blessing in adversity." I believe it since now I can sympathize with all Lyme patients and understand from my personal battle with the terrorist and what it is like to be on the front line against this unbelievably rabid tick-borne disease.

So how am I doing today? Not 100% cured, but doing much better than a few years ago. I am certain of one thing - there is no one treatment that works for all. Every individual needs to be individually treated depending on his/her history and tolerances to different medications and methods.

Yes, the fight goes on...

The final episode of this fight will be forthcoming as we the people put our shoulders to the task of awakening the masses including professionals to recognize the problem and making a difference in battling the 'terrorist within' by education, action, and advocacy, both individually and collectively with the hope that State and Federal authorities will finally see the need and lend a major hand to win the battle and overcome the 'terrorist within' before it is too late!

May God bless you as you continue to increase your knowledge about the "terorist within" - you will help yourself, your family, and even your busy doctor to unravel many of the strange and sometimes alarming symptoms of Lyme and its co-infections!

I wish you the best as you search for the answers!

Your Lyme Doc,

Gordon A. Gilkes, MD, MPH

You may obtain additional copies of this book as well as further updates, news, and inspiration in this fight against Lyme disease by visiting my daughter's website:

www.LymeFacts.com

or emailing

Lucia@lymefacts.com

ACKNOWLEDGEMENTS

❃ ❃ ❃

I would like to thank my brother Michael who helped edit the manuscript, bringing both his poetry and playwriting skills to bear on the task. He's a doctor of Literature (University of Kent at Canterbury, England) and has also worked as a qualified pharmacist, so his contribution was powered by both a literary and a practical medical interest.

I would also like to thank my nephew Richard Hardinge who assisted in the editing of the manuscript and also provided ideas and graphic designs for the cover. Richard lives in Manitoba, Canada where he uses his skills in computer technology to trouble-shoot problems and keep the Brandon Hospital's computer systems functioning smoothly.

Special thanks go out to Jim Wilson, CEO of the *Canadian Lyme Foundation* for taking the time to read the first 60 pages of the manuscript and making suggestions for correcting some of the information presented. Jim knows from personal experience what Lyme disease is all about and has himself successfully battled the "the terrorist within". His is a powerful voice for the thousands of Lyme patients on both sides of the Canadian/United States border. I have learned a great deal from the www.canlyme.com web pages and I encourage anyone who wants to know more about Lyme disease to make that web page a must. There is a growing Lyme epidemic which government medical departments and private medical societies ignore at their (and our) peril.

My heartfelt thanks to Arna Lucia Gilkes. Her support has been unstinting both as a registered nurse and a dear wife of more than 50 years. We both have had close and personal experiences with many Lyme patients of different ages and widely different symptoms. She and I were both involved in a "preceptorship" offered via ILADS (International Lyme and Associated Diseases Society) and sponsored by a Turn the Corner Foundation grant. This was a highlight for both of us in 2007.

Thanks are also due to the many friends and family members whose encouragement was invaluable. These include my daughter Lucia Ann Tiffany, Laure and Art Andreas, Art and Melody Johnson, Uchi Pines Institute in Alabama and Marsha Hardinge and Maureen Yates, my two sisters who encouraged me constantly when I needed a boost to keep working on the book.

Last but not least, I must thank all the many Lyme patients with whom I consulted and encouraged to get tested for Lyme disease via IgeneX lab in Palo Alto California. It was their plight that really inspired me to start writing this book in the first place and so perhaps help thousands of infected persons understand their strange, sometimes bizarre, and often inexplicable symptoms.